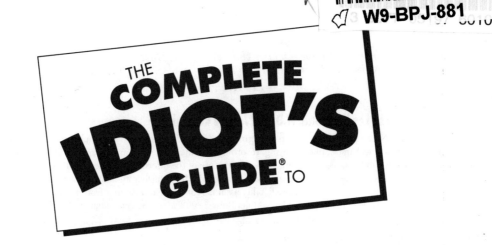

THE COMPLETE IDIOT'S GUIDE® TO

Food Allergies

by Lee H. Freund, M.D and Jeanne Rejaunier

ALPHA

A member of Penguin Group (USA) Inc.

Dedicated to my wife, Elaine, and our children, Mark, David, and Karen, who have always been and continue to be a source of pride, strength, and love.

—Lee H. Freund

Most Alpha books are available at special quantity discounts for bulk purchases for sales promotions, premiums, fund-raising, or educational use. Special books, or book excerpts, can also be created to fit specific needs.

For details, write: Special Markets, Alpha Books, 375 Hudson Street, New York, NY 10014.

Publisher: *Marie Butler-Knight*
Product Manager: *Phil Kitchel*
Senior Managing Editor: *Jennifer Chisholm*
Acquisitions Editor: *Mikal Belicove*
Development Editor: *Michael Koch*
Production Editor: *Megan Douglass*
Copy Editor: *Drew Patty*
Illustrator: *Chris Eliopoulos*
Cover/Book Designer: *Trina Wurst*
Indexer: *Angie Bess*
Layout/Proofreading: *Rebecca Harmon, John Etchison*

Contents at a Glance

Appendixes

Contents

Foreword

Food allergies can be one of life's major health challenges. For the truly allergic person, every meal and morsel of food must be questioned or scrutinized to prevent an allergic reaction. For highly sensitive individuals, even one bite of the wrong food can be lethal if not treated properly and promptly.

I was diagnosed with a multitude of food allergies back when I was in diapers. My mother would feed me a meal and it would quickly come right back out one way or another. My poor mother had to figure out what to feed me when I reacted to over 60 different foods. Can you imagine what life was like with a child who had negative reactions to so many different foods? Some caused minimal distress like nasal congestion, while other foods or food combinations triggered stomachache, chest pains, vomiting, diarrhea, itchy mouth, scratchy throat, raspy voice, and red eyes. Severe reactions included a combination of the above and a terrifying asthma attack. Imagine watching your small child struggle to gasp for breath. How helpless my parents must have felt. There were dozens of nights where we would race off to the ER to be given a lifesaving dose of adrenaline. Our family physician finally showed my father how to inject the lifesaving serum into my arm to prevent the frequent middle-of-the-night emergency room journeys.

The Complete Idiot's Guide to Food Allergies would have been a tremendous resource for my parents when I was initially diagnosed with food allergies. It would have answered countless questions, helping them to better understand what it means to suffer from food allergies. This book can help you to learn more about your food allergy-related problems, and can help you to understand whether your reactions call for a trip to the physician's office for a professional diagnosis or to the emergency room for immediate treatment. If you or a family member have recently been tested and diagnosed with food allergies, this book thoroughly covers many aspects of food allergies you will want to know about. The authors even provide up-to-date information on recent allergy breakthroughs, as well as tips to help you eat safely when dining out.

The Complete Idiot's Guide to Food Allergies also offers a detailed description of how food allergens affect your body's immune system. The book even goes so far as to explore old-world alternative healing therapies that traditional doctors may or may not support.

Knowledge is power. Read this book so you can better understand how food allergens affect you or your loved one. If you or someone in your family has food allergies, or even if you suspect that they do, then reading this book will provide a wealth of important and timely information.

Joanne Schlosser

President, Food Allergy Awareness Institute

Joanne Schlosser is president of The Food Allergy Awareness Institute, a Scottsdale, Arizona-based organization that works with the foodservice industry to provide education to safely serve guests with food allergies. Hotels, restaurants, resorts, caterers, culinary schools, and others have learned how to meet the needs of those with severe food allergies. Schlosser is the author of *Serving the Allergic Guest: Increasing Profit, Loyalty and Safety* and an online newsletter, *Food Allergy News You Can Use*. For more information on the Food Allergy Awareness Institute, visit www.fdalrgy.com.

Introduction

This book may be called *The Complete Idiot's Guide to Food Allergies,* but it takes a smart person like you to want to fully understand what your food allergy, food intolerance, or other adverse food problems are all about, and discover how to do something positive about the situation. Reading this book will enable you to take the bull by the horns and start taking those all-important, positive steps forward that have heretofore eluded you.

The Complete Idiot's Guide to Food Allergies covers the whole spectrum of food-allergic symptoms as well as those that mimic food allergies. We give you the big picture, with lots of details and tidbits that can not only educate you, but provide you with the confidence to overcome obstacles and live a safe and healthy lifestyle. Along the way, you'll find answers to the following questions and more:

- What are the odds of you having a child with food allergies if you are/are not allergic yourself?

- Can a person be allergic to alcohol?

- What are the safest medications for pregnant women?

- Is it true a person can die from kissing someone who's just eaten peanuts?

- What should you do if you're accidentally exposed to the wrong foods?

- What are the most common food-allergic symptoms?

- How can you tell if you're really allergic, or if you actually have food intolerance?

- When should you consult a doctor for adverse reactions to food?

- Is it true allergies are different in different parts of the country and the world?

- Can eating rhubarb pie actually kill you?

- Can a person have a food allergy and not know it?

- How serious are food allergies? Can one die from them?

- In cooking, what ingredients can be substituted for the ones you're allergic to?

- What common supermarket foods contain hidden allergens?

Read on to find out the answers to these questions, and many more!

What You'll Learn in This Book

The *Complete Idiot's Guide to Food Allergies* is divided into five parts.

Part 1, "Face the Enemy," teaches you how to distinguish a food allergy from a food intolerance. It also introduces the eight foods that account for 80 to 90 percent of all food-allergic reactions. In this part, you'll also get a historical overview of allergy research and a closer look at the chemical processes in your body that are at the very root of food-allergic problems.

Part 2, "Bring on the Food," helps you understand the various corners from which foods can stage an attack: foods that contain histamine, foods with toxic agents, and contaminated foods all play their part, causing gastroesophageal reflux (GERD), laryngopharyngeal reflux (LPR), heartburn, and hiatal hernia—these are all symptoms which are often mistaken for food allergies. The part concludes with a close-up on the major foods that can trigger an allergic reaction.

Part 3, "A Visit to Your Allergist," focuses on what to expect when you consult an allergist. What happens during a physical examination? What are the signs of a good diagnostician? What's the best way of testing for a food allergy? You'll hear about the many types of antihistamines—the pros and cons of how each works, the symptoms they treat, and side effects you should be aware of—as well as other allergy medication.

Part 4, "The Allergic Family," looks at food allergy in babies and children and adverse reactions from foods in older people. It also covers allergies in pets, and provides tips on smart shopping for safe food. Find out how to spot hidden ingredients on food labels and how to make your restaurant dining safer and stress-free both at home and abroad.

Part 5, "Alternative and Complementary Help," begins by examining quack modalities which claim to diagnose, treat, and "cure" food allergies. You'll learn what's safe and what's dangerous and which treatments, herbs, vitamins, minerals, and supplements may possibly help adverse food symptoms. The information and content presented in this part are only for your general information and should not be relied on as medical advice. The authors and publisher do not endorse or recommend the treatments discussed in this part. If you experience allergy or other health problems, we encourage you to seek out your own trained medical practitioner first for advice, diagnosis, and treatment regarding any medical condition.

At the end of the book, you'll find two appendixes with resources for additional information and a glossary.

How to Use This Book

No, you don't have to begin at the beginning, you don't have to digest every word, and you don't have to plow through to the end of this book, either. Just find what you want to read. Glance through the table of contents or give the book the "flick test"; pick out what interests you and go for it. Because *The Complete Idiot's Guide to Food Allergies* covers the entire gamut of adverse food reactions, there's something here for everyone. As a discriminating reader, you'll know not to bother spending time on the parts that don't apply to you ... if you're in your late 20s, single, and eating wheat makes you break out in hives, you might not be interested in reading material about babies, children, older adults, or lactose intolerance, for example. But rest assured, no stone has been left unturned. It's all here, within these covers. Trust us.

Extras

For your reading pleasure, *The Complete Idiot's Guide to Food Allergies* contains a variety of boxed sidebars. They'll all add to your knowledge in some way, but each does it differently. Here's the rundown:

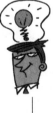 **Bet You Didn't Know**

Okay, maybe you do know, but we're betting you don't, so we're pointing out interesting assorted information we think you might like to hear about.

 Med Meaning

These notes provide definitions of terms used in the text. Read them and you'll know what the experts are talking about.

 Skulls and Bones

Watch out! This note advises caution; read it carefully, so you don't make any mistakes.

 Timely Tip

These notes offer tidbits of advice, geared to specific points.

Acknowledgments

No book is ever a solo effort. We would like to thank the many people and organizations whose expertise was made available for this book. Special thanks go to: our erstwhile acquisitions editor Eric Heagy, who started the ball rolling; acquisitions editor Mikal Belicove, who on short notice kept everything moving so smoothly; our talented and perceptive development editor Michael Koch and technical editor Joanne Schlosser; our enterprising agent BK Nelson, together with ever-vigilant support staff John Benson. Those whose contributions are also highly appreciated include Stella Fiore, Fanny Maltz, Robert F. Joseph, M.D., Howard Harrison, Ellen King, Lisa Fox, Dennis Fox, M.D., Johanna G. Sherman, Frances C. Walloch-Staros, C.T.A., Judy Whitney, Gerald H. Vind, and most of all … thanks to the steady and ongoing love, help, and support of Elaine Freund.

Special Thanks to the Technical Reviewer

The Complete Idiot's Guide to Food Allergies was reviewed by an expert who double-checked the accuracy of what you'll learn here, to help us ensure that this book gives you everything you need to know about food allergies. Special thanks are extended to Joanne Schlosser.

Trademarks

All terms mentioned in this book that are known to be or are suspected of being trademarks or service marks have been appropriately capitalized. Alpha Books and Penguin Group (USA) Inc. cannot attest to the accuracy of this information. Use of a term in this book should not be regarded as affecting the validity of any trademark or service mark.

In Memoriam

The author, Dr. Lee H. Freund, passed away unexpectedly after the completion of this book. Dr. Freund was a compassionate pediatrician and allergist who cared deeply about the education people received on issues surrounding food allergies and related intolerances. Dr. Freund's presence in and contributions to the medical community will be sorely missed.

Part 1

Face the Enemy

The only way to conquer the enemy is to face the threat head-on. The first part of this book introduces you to the world of adverse food reactions. Beginning with the basics, this section looks at food allergies—what causes them, who gets them, why, and how. You'll also learn to distinguish between true allergic reactions to food and food intolerance, when an allergic reaction is dangerous, and when allergies will and won't disappear.

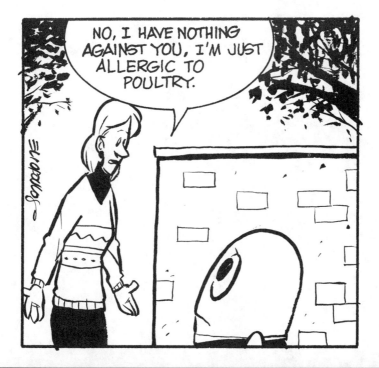

Introducing Food Allergies and Food Intolerance

In This Chapter

- ◆ Learn to distinguish between a food allergy and food intolerance
- ◆ Find out who is prone to have food allergies and why
- ◆ Identify the symptoms of an allergic reaction to foods
- ◆ Sort through the different views on why allergies are on the rise

There are at least two good reasons to learn about allergies. One is that there seems to be an increase in the number of allergy problems in the general population. Another, even better one is that you or a family member may have allergy problems and want to get help.

The number of people reported with allergy symptoms is growing; in some reports this number is almost twice as many as those reported 10 to 20 years ago. The reason for this can be found in a number of directions. We will explore the methods of reporting allergies. Maybe there are the same number of cases relative to the growth in the population, but they are more accurately identified and reported. Other areas to look at are the effect of moving from rural to urban areas, modernization with exposure to pollutants, and diet changes from home-cooked to commercially prepared foods. There are many other theories involving the environment in our homes, at work, and outside. Some feel that there are toxic chemicals in the building materials of our homes and/ or workplaces. Another group feels that the food and water supply is contaminated.

For whatever reason, we are seeing more people with symptoms of inhalant and food allergies. To help you to learn about the latter, we will begin with an understanding of what a true allergic reaction is. Some of these symptoms are true food allergies; more commonly they are the result of food intolerance, which is actually a more common occurrence. This is a key difference and must be understood to get help for the symptoms. Food intolerance can look and feel like an allergy but is from other causes. Once identified, it is easier to recognize and hopefully relieve the problem. The chapter will begin to answer these questions: Why do allergies occur? Why are we seeing more people with allergies? Who is affected? What are the causes? Finally, we will be looking to the future and what is in store with exciting new approaches to a very annoying and sometimes fatal problem.

Allergies in Theory

Experience has shown us that about 20 percent of the population have allergies. Recently that number is being estimated upward to 35 percent and even higher when all allergies, both inhalant and food, are included. Some researchers in university teaching centers attribute this surge in allergy sufferers to environmental changes. Theories state that there's more air contamination and more exposure to harmful chemicals in the environment. It is hypothesized that pollutants react on the immune system through changes in the DNA of cells, thus possibly increasing their reactivity. This is a theoretical explanation for the observation that there seem to be fewer allergies reported in rural areas than urban areas.

Other clinicians feel that we have become more urbanized, which is causing more problems with allergies and other respiratory disorders.

Still another group of clinicians argues that the above factors may be part of the problem, but also that the public and medical caregivers are being educated to recognize an allergy as a cause more frequently. They say that the problem existed all along, except that previously, insufficient attention was drawn to it. Therefore, the reported incidence of allergies in a group studied may really be better and more accurate recognition of allergy as a cause of some problem. An example is colic in infants that may really be a food allergy, and summer colds that may actually be "hay fever."

At any rate, the prevalence of food allergies is growing, and in all probability will continue to grow, along with all other allergic diseases. Research indicates that the number of people with allergies is increasing in the West, but not in nonindustrialized countries. Paradoxically, some researchers feel it seems that the fewer germs we have floating around in our environment and in our systems, the more our immune system will gravitate to allergens. They theorize that as natural immunity decreases, the immune system starts working less efficiently. In fact, some recent studies seem to indicate that growing up in a large family or spending much of one's early childhood in a daycare center actually decreases the likelihood of developing an allergy. But for many members of the medical community, the evidence of a connection between environmental factors and allergies is still inclusive.

Understanding Allergic Reactions to Food

Eating is an enjoyable part of life at best, and something we can't avoid at worst—so eating a food that makes us ill is a serious problem. Symptoms of an allergic reaction to food can result in anything from a mild nuisance to a serious, life-threatening situation. Most allergic reactions occur immediately after eating the offending food, and may range anywhere from itchy eyes to severe respiratory problems. Other allergic reactions may take hours to develop. Some examples of this are people severely allergic to peanuts or tree nuts who may react with hives, swollen eyes, and/or breathing problems within minutes of eating even small amounts. At the other extreme, some reactions may not appear until 48 to 72 hours later. This more commonly happens with medications or vitamins and supplements.

Skulls and Bones

For some people, food allergies cause only a slight itch, gas, or an upset stomach; in others, even touching or inhaling the wrong food can lead to serious illness or death.

Zooming In on the Offending Food

In a nutshell, allergic reactions are the result of a built-in protective mechanism of your body, not unlike the type of protection you get on a computer when installing anti-virus software. If a computer virus in the form of an infected e-mail or document reaches your PC or Mac, your anti-virus software intercepts the potentially harmful intruder and neutralizes it. Likewise, your body is equipped with an immune system programmed to recognize harmful substances that get into your blood system or organs. If a harmful substance or *allergen* enters your body, the immune system reacts through a system of plasma proteins called *immunoglobulins* that search out and destroy the intruder. (For more details on this process, see Chapter 2.)

However, for an allergic reaction to occur, you must first become sensitized to an offending *food allergen* or protein. One or more encounters with the allergen are required before sensitization develops. The first exposure "programs" your immune system to recognize and react in a certain way when encountering this allergen. Subsequent exposures result in your allergic reaction to that particular food protein. In essence, your immune system reacts to this allergen as a threatening foreign substance and primes your body's defenses against it by releasing *histamine* and other chemicals called *mediators*, which in turn trigger symptoms of an allergic reaction in your nose, throat, lungs, skin, or gastrointestinal tract. When this occurs, you have developed what doctors call an *immediate hypersensitivity* reaction to the offending food.

Med Meaning

A **food allergen** is a protein within food that usually is not broken down either by cooking or by stomach acids or enzymes. Instead, it survives to reach the gastrointestinal lining, reacting with so-called IgE antibodies on cells that might be in the gut lining, or passes through the lining into the bloodstream and reacts with IgE to release **mediators** that call other cells to help. In either case, there is release of chemical mediators, including histamine. These travel to the target organ (skin, nose, eyes lungs, and so on) and create the symptoms. **Histamine** is a chemical released by cells of the immune system called *mast cells*. This chemical is largely responsible for producing the symptoms associated with allergic reactions.

To Be or Not to Be a Food Allergy

Often, people who experience symptoms such as a cough, runny nose, cramping, and so on after eating food, automatically draw the conclusion that their discomfort must be the result of an allergic reaction to that food. However, that may not be the case. A condition called *food intolerance* is frequently mistaken for a food allergy. The difference between the two is how the body handles the offending food. Although both of these conditions may share similar symptoms, a food allergy is an immune system response. Food intolerance occurs when the digestive tract reacts adversely to a food. This reaction does not involve immunoglobulin E or IgE antibodies (see Med Meaning sidebar earlier), which are prevalent in allergic reactions. One example is a problem in which the body lacks the enzyme to "digest" the lactose in milk. This type of intolerance is called *lactose intolerance*. Exposure to toxins in our foods or in our food supply is not an allergic reaction, but truly a toxic or type of "poison" reaction which involves other defense mechanisms. These toxins react on the tissues of the body directly. Examples of this would be toxins in some shellfish during certain seasons of the year. Once again, this shows how complicated it is to find the exact cause of food-related problems.

Food intolerance is a far more prevalent problem than food allergy, affecting nearly everybody at some point. If you consume a food and end up with an adverse reaction, you can safely assume that your reactions are produced either by the immune system (as a result of food allergy) or by the gastrointestinal system (as a result of food intolerance). Together with your doctor, you'll need to determine the true nature of your condition— food allergy or intolerance—before you can take the appropriate next steps toward an allergy-free and healthier life.

Skulls and Bones

Self-diagnosis can be dangerous, even fatal. Always seek medical advice before treating an allergy.

Blame It on Your Genes ... and the Environment

Scientific research has shown that genetics plays an important role in allergic reactions to food. Research also has shown that repeated exposure to allergens can begin sensitizing the susceptible person, and that repeated exposure to the same foods, particularly in large quantities, can trigger allergic reactions, as seen in the high prevalence of fish allergies among Scandinavians, and rice and soy allergies among the Japanese. The culprit in these reactions is the protein part of a food, more specifically the size and shape of the protein molecule in both raw and cooked food.

The Straight Skinny

The chance of an individual forming an allergy against food is inherited. Generally, such people come from families in which allergies are common. In these people, certain foods will trigger the cells of the immune system to produce a series of reactions that will cause allergic symptoms. It has been suggested that exposure to these foods in early infancy is a big factor in developing allergies.

Some people are born with the inherited tendency to have allergies. That's only half the story. What you're exposed to in your environment both before and after birth will determine whether you actually develop allergy symptoms. You may be ripe to react but never be put in a place where you will react. An example of this would be an infant whose mother and father both have bad allergies to pollen. If the baby is breast-fed for 6 months or more and the mother avoids eating highly allergenic foods during that time, there is a very low chance that the infant will have allergies to those foods. Even better, if the foods are kept out of the baby's diet until 12 months, there is still less chance of a food allergy to these allergens for the first three years.

It Runs in the Family

Most allergy patients have parents, aunts, uncles, or grandparents who suffer from some form of allergy. The trick is to pinpoint who in your family might have had allergies that were unrecognized. For example, Grandpa always had bronchitis every summer. Mom or Dad has a cough or cold every spring. A family member having breathing problems every Christmas may not have a cold, but an allergic reaction to the Christmas tree. Summer or spring colds could be pollen allergies, which also run in families. This knowledge is important when we want to advise which newborn should be kept on a strict diet, as already mentioned.

If both your parents have allergies, you have approximately a 75 percent chance of being allergic. If one parent is allergic, or if you have relatives on one side with food allergies, you have a 30 to 40 percent chance of developing an allergy in general. If neither parent has an apparent allergy, your chance still is 10 to 15 percent.

> **Skulls and Bones** ___
>
> If you suspect you have a food allergy, you must seek medical help. Because a food allergy may be potentially dangerous, it should never go untreated.

Food allergy occurs in about 2 percent to 8 percent of the general population. As you can see, these are only approximations and a numbers game. The important thing here is that true food allergy is less frequent than other allergies.

Just the Facts, Ma'am

Allergies, not just food allergies, can strike anyone at any time of life. A baby can be born allergic, or a heretofore unafflicted adult can develop an allergy out of the blue. A food allergy can even be caused by foods that had been previously eaten without a hitch.

Some people are prone to just one type of allergy, while others may get a mixture. An allergic person can be allergic to inhalants such as pollen or mites, etc. Some of these people are also allergic to a variety of foods.

It's also possible to have had allergies for a length of time without even realizing it. In some cases, one might "outgrow" the allergy; this happens when the person develops a tolerance to certain foods. It has been noted that some infants that have cow's milk or egg allergies early in life may develop a tolerance to these foods as they grow older. Or an allergy may start to disappear, only to reappear later. Some people may subsequently develop additional sensitivities, and in yet others, the sensitivity may diminish or disappear altogether. Immunologists have even suggested introducing minute amounts of the allergen to allow the body to learn to accept it, sort of like a self-vaccination in steps.

Unfortunately, for some people food allergies are a serious matter. For them, just a taste or even a touch of the wrong foods can set off a chain reaction that, in the most severe cases, takes only minutes to culminate in an often-fatal condition known as *anaphylaxis*, which is discussed in detail in Chapter 3.

Victim List

Here are some food allergy-related facts that may surprise you:

- Scientists estimate that only 1 percent to 2 percent of all adults—between 6 and 7 million people—suffer from true food allergies, although an estimated 40 to 50 million Americans have allergies.

- Three percent to 8 percent of children under age six have adverse reactions to ingested foods; between 2 percent and 6 percent have confirmed food allergies.

- Many children outgrow their hypersensitivity to foods by age 10. However, allergies to peanuts, tree nuts, and shellfish do not usually go away.

- One out of three people say they either have a food allergy or intolerance, or that they modify the family diet because a family member is allergic or intolerant.

- Unlike allergies, food intolerance generally intensifies with age.

- Many people suffer from lactose intolerance without realizing it, and remain in distress unnecessarily.

- Only about 7 percent to 10 percent of Caucasians are lactose intolerant, 85 percent to 95 percent of Asians have lactose intolerance, while 60 percent to 75 percent of Blacks, 40 percent to 50 percent of Mediterranean and Hispanic people, and 10 percent to 15 percent of Northern Europeans are affected.

Signs of an Allergic Reaction

Symptoms, frequency, and severity of food allergies differ from one person to another. Mildly allergic persons may suffer only a slightly runny nose or sneezing, while those who are highly allergic may experience severe, life-threatening reactions.

The most common symptoms of food allergies are …

- **Skin reactions.** Itchy red rash, hives, and eczema.

- **Stomach and intestinal reactions.** Abdominal pain and bloating, diarrhea, vomiting, gas/flatulence, and cramps.

◆ **Nose, throat, and lung reactions.** Runny nose, sneezing, watery and/or itchy eyes, coughing, wheezing, and shortness of breath.

Some six dozen or more medical conditions are often attributed to or associated with food allergies, although they have nothing to do with true food allergies, including …

◆ **Respiratory conditions.** Hay fever, bronchitis, ear infections, sinusitis, rhinitis, laryngitis, sore throat, and hoarseness.

◆ **Digestive conditions.** Gastroenteritis, irritable bowel syndrome, celiac disease, inflammatory bowel disease, and constipation.

◆ **Cerebral conditions.** Headaches, dizziness, sleep disorders, learning disabilities, and irritability.

◆ **Skin-related conditions.** Dermatitis, angioedema, hives, and rashes.

◆ **Conditions related to other body systems.** Arthritis myalgia, urinary problems, conjunctivitis, edema, diabetes, and premenstrual syndrome.

Vittles Most Foul

Some 160 foods have been reported to cause allergic reactions in humans. However, although one could be allergic to any food—such as fruits, vegetables, and meats—these are not as common as the following eight foods, which account for 80 percent to 90 percent of all food allergy reactions:

◆ Milk

◆ Eggs

◆ Peanuts

◆ Tree nuts (almond, walnut, cashew, and so on)

◆ Fish

◆ Shellfish

◆ Soy

◆ Wheat

In the past it was felt that some people are also sensitive to food additives, food coloring, monosodium glutamate, or salicylates, which are aspirin-like substances occurring naturally in foods such as dried and berry fruits, oranges, grapes, almonds, peppermint, honey, many herbs, tea, wine, and port. Currently there is a question as to the accuracy of this.

You should also know that foods, just like people, come in families, and knowing the food family each food is a part of will help you identify the food group that causes you discomfort, and thus help you avoid reactions by eliminating all foods in that group. For example, people allergic to shrimp are usually also allergic to lobster and crab, all of which belong to the family known as crustaceans. (For a complete list of food families, skip ahead to Chapter 6.)

Last, but not least, you should know that some foods cross-react with certain plants, for example melons and weeds. Many times patients have a history of having an itchy mouth and throat when eating melons. When they consult an allergist who runs some allergy tests on them, it turns out they are allergic to weeds. (Foods that cross-react with plants and other foods are discussed in Chapter 3.)

A very small number of people with food allergies are even sensitive to the food while it is being cooked. In the process of cooking peanuts, for example, minute particles of the food are released. This has also been reported with exposure to cooking fish. A very allergic person has been reported to have an allergic reaction by just inhaling these particles. Many years ago when this was first reported, it was called *osmoles*.

Bet You Didn't Know

Almost half of children outgrow food allergies after the age of 3 to 5, and 75 percent by age 7, especially for dairy products and eggs; however, sensitivities to peanuts, nuts, fish and shellfish tend to be lifelong. Adults usually do not lose their allergies.

A Farewell to Allergies?

Can anybody really ever outgrow allergies? The good news is it looks like some children develop a tolerance to certain foods early in life, before they grow up to be teenagers. Do they really *lose* the allergy? The bad news is no; but they can become tolerant to some food, or the intestinal tract matures and blocks some of the problem foods from getting into the circulatory system. This again seems to relate to how much exposure happens as we get older.

Of course, you can get a variety of prescriptions for food allergy relief. You can also choose from a variety of alternative remedies that purport to help people seeking relief from their allergies. Beware, however, for many of these alternatives have not shown consistently positive results in clinical tests; so instead of treating your allergies, they may only burn a hole in your wallet. The best treatment that money can't buy is still recognizing the food that bothers you, and then staying as far away from the offender as you can. In order to get there, however, you first have to consult an allergist who can diagnose the problem and help you become educated about your condition.

What about allergy shots? Unfortunately, the problem can't be helped with injections at the present time. Currently, some researchers think there is a way; some are talking about future treatments that may offer this alternative. So all we can do at this juncture is to stay tuned, cheer the researchers on, and keep our hopes up. Most recently, there have been reports of research teams with new and exciting ways of handling food allergy. Later we will go into the details. These methods include getting shots of a material that blocks the IgE protein in the blood needed to create an allergic reaction. Another possibility is a shot program in which the allergen, the food or pollen, is joined to part of another harmless protein, hopefully to make the person less sensitive to the food that causes the allergy.

In the next chapter, we will delve into the history of allergies, and also dive into the bloodstream to see what is the root cause of allergies.

Bet You Didn't Know

Unfortunately, at the present time there is no cure per se for food allergies; avoiding the offending food or foods is the only sure way to totally prevent an allergic reaction and bring your allergy problem under control so that it will cease to bother you.

The Least You Need to Know

  - ♦ Food allergies affect only a small percentage of people, more commonly in developed countries.

  - ♦ The majority of food allergies are caused by only eight foods.

  - ♦ Allergic symptoms are varied, affecting the respiratory and gastrointestinal systems, as well as the skin and other organs.

  - ♦ Confusing an allergy with food intolerance, many people falsely believe they are allergic.

  - ♦ While some cases of food allergy are not life-threatening, others can be potentially dangerous and require medical treatment.

Understanding Allergic Reactions

In This Chapter

- ◆ Take a whirlwind tour of allergy research through the ages
- ◆ Look inside the protective mechanisms of the immune system
- ◆ Identify the steps involved in an allergic reaction
- ◆ Understand the four types of immune reactions

This chapter looks at how the knowledge of food allergies developed over the ages, how the ancients suffered the same adverse food reactions we do today, even if they didn't call it a "food allergy," and also notes some of the landmarks in allergy research, particularly over the past 100 years. Today, we know that allergic reactions are the result of an overreacting immune system, so it's important to understand basic facts about the body's built-in protection system, about the process of sensitization, about antibodies and allergens, and about what can go wrong with this system, and why.

Allergies Yesterday and Today

Although food allergies appear to be an increasingly common problem among Western populations, it is not a new phenomenon. Since ancient times, people have been aware that the consumption of presumably harmless substances can cause serious health problems for some people. As early as 400 B.C.E., the Greek physician Hippocrates (c. 460–c. 370 B.C.E.), also known as the father of modern medicine, observed that some of his patients got sick to their stomachs and broke out in rashes after drinking milk, and others showed similar symptoms or went into shock after consuming shellfish. However, it wasn't until the nineteenth century that scientists, through experimental observations, sought to describe in scientific terms what Hippocrates and those who followed in his footsteps had been observing for centuries—the body's immune system reacting to offending substances in foods and the environment.

In 1839, the French physiologist François Magendie (1783–1855), while investigating the effects of substances on living organisms, created allergylike symptoms in animals, and found that animals sensitized to egg white by injection died after a subsequent injection.

By the mid-1800s, the condition we identify today as hay fever had been traced to grass and wheat pollens, thanks to the pioneering work of Charles Harrison Blackley (1820–1900), a surgeon from Manchester, England.

The idea of cells being directly involved in defending the human body against potentially harmful substances was first suggested by the Russian biologist and Nobel laureate Ilya Metchnikoff (1845–1916) in 1884. Metchnikoff, aware that single-cell organisms took in food by *phagocytosis* and released debris by *exocytosis*, suggested that phagocytic cells in vertebrates might operate in a similar fashion. Like macrophages, phagocytic cells are an early defense against invading bacteria.

Med Meaning

Phagocytosis refers to the process by which white blood cells engulf material and enclose it within a vacuole in the cytoplasm (protoplasm), everything between the cell membrane and the nuclear envelope. **Exocytosis** is the mechanism by which cells release molecules such as proteins.

In 1901, French scientist Charles Richet (1850–1935) coined the word *anaphylaxis* to designate the sensitivity developed by an organism after being given an injection of protein or toxin. Twelve years later, Richet was awarded the Nobel Prize for his research on anaphylaxis.

The word *allergy*—which comes from the Greek *allos*, meaning "changed or altered state," and *ergon* meaning "reaction or reactivity"—was coined in 1906 by the Viennese physician Baron Clemens Peter Freiherr von Pirquet (1874–1929) to describe an "altered response" in his patients' bodies after food intake. Noting that patients receiving antitoxin serum developed symptoms of fever and rash, von Pirquet discussed the relationship between hypersensitivity (or the onset of allergic reactions) and immunity, and also developed a new theory about the formation of antibodies. Von Pirquet also coined the term *allergen*, the substance responsible for the altered reaction.

The same year that von Pirquet coined the term *allergy*, German physician Alfred Wolff-Eisner (1877–1948) invented the terms *pollen disease* and *pollen sensitivity*, suggesting that hay fever might be a form of hypersensitivity or anaphylaxis in the nose. Four years later, American physiologist Samuel Meltzer (1851–1920) made the connection between asthma and allergy.

In 1910, while experimenting with allergic diseases, the British scientist Sir Henry Dale (1875–1968) identified *histamine*—a substance released by the body's tissues, as a key "mediator" in the body's allergic response.

It was discovered that histamine, when placed on guinea pig tissue, would cause blood vessels to dilate and to leak out serum and white blood cells. If this process happens in the nose, congestion and a runny nose result; in the skin, this reaction causes itching and welts; in the lungs, it causes congestion, swelling, shortness of breath, or even wheezing. This explained that only one substance—that which was in the serum—could lead to most of the symptoms called an allergic reaction. Later additional substances called mediators were discovered to play a part in the full allergic reaction.

The next step was to chemically produce artificial histamine in a test tube. In 1937, Bover and Staub accidentally discovered antagonists to histamine. By 1942, safe forms for human use of antihistamines were perfected.

The first study of genetic predisposition to allergy, published by Robert Cooke (1857–1936) and Albert Vander Veer (1878–1959) in 1916, concluded that inheritance is a factor in human sensitization. The study also suggested that sensitization is inherited as an unusual capacity to react to foreign proteins. Cooke and Vander Veer called the protein factor involved *atopic reagin*, and coined the term *atopy* to designate those human hypersensitivity conditions that are genetically inherited.

 Med Meaning

The word **atopic** comes from the Greek word *a* ("negative") + *topos* ("place"), meaning "without a place." The atopic conditions asthma, hay fever, and eczema (atopic dermatitis) were classified as "strange diseases," all of which were inherited via a dominant gene.

Further study of atopic hypersensitivity revealed that a common immune mechanism—a single antibody species then known as *reaginic antibody*—was responsible for some of the typical manifestations of atopic conditions, and that an inherited tendency to produce excessive amounts of the reaginic antibody is one characteristic of atopic individuals (otherwise known as allergy sufferers).

Clinical Allergy Daddy-O

Carl Prausnitz (1876–1963) is remembered as the discoverer of the Prausnitz-Küstner reaction and, more important, as the "father of clinical allergies."

Working in Germany in the early part of the twentieth century, Prausnitz and an associate—both hay fever sufferers—experimented on themselves, and through injections, developed severe asthma and hives. Later, in 1921, Prausnitz and his colleague Heinz Küstner demonstrated a *passive transfer* of allergies.

Med Meaning

Passive transfer is a test in which serum from a person known to be allergic to a certain food (such as fish) is injected under the skin of a nonallergic person; 24 to 48 hours later if the nonallergic person eats fish, the area of skin where the injection was made will form a hive. Thus the reagin, specific IgE, is passively transferred to the skin of the second, nonallergic person.

Prausnitz and Küstner were each allergic to different substances. Küstner suffered from an allergy to fish, the tiniest taste of which would make his mouth swell. The two scientists injected themselves with small amounts of each other's blood. The next day fish extract was injected. A typical red wheal and erythematic reaction—the redness of the skin—that emerged on Prausnitz's arm after local administration of the allergen showed that sensitivity to particular substances could be transferred via *serum* from an allergic person to a nonallergic one.

Med Meaning

Serum is the part of the blood without cells. Passing serum from one patient to another is very dangerous, because of the possibility of transferring AIDS or hepatitis.

This discovery of the passive transfer of hypersensitivity, which was of immense importance to the understanding of hay fever, asthma, eczema, and food allergies, served to propel Prausnitz to the stature of an international figure.

Food Allergies Under the Microscope

Prausnitz and Küstner were not alone in their efforts to isolate and expose the reaginic antibodies responsible for allergic reactions to foods. For the next 30 years, many doctors conducted similar experiments with similar results, particularly involving allergens such as egg and milk. In 1905, British psychiatrist Francis Hare published the book *The Food Factor in Disease*. In 1921, William Duke reported cases in which three allergens—eggs, milk, and wheat—produced stomach upsets.

In 1925, when Dr. Erwin Pulay published a book on eczema and hives, scientists were making diagnoses of allergic responses in sensitized subjects to foods.

Dr. Arthur Coca (1875–1959), a Professor at Cornell in the 1930s and a co-founder of the *Journal of Immunology*, researched a number of allergic responses to ingested substances. Dr. Coca has been credited as having demonstrated the role of heredity in food allergy sufferers. (Coca is also the inventor of the Coca Pulse Test, which was widely used at one time, later became incorporated in the Rinkel test, and now is mostly discredited in the conventional allergy field.)

In the late 1930s, Dr. Herbert Rinkel, a practicing allergist, had a severe allergic response. For many years before this, Rinkel had suffered from fatigue, headaches, and runny nose. Suspecting an egg allergy, Rinkel consumed six raw eggs in a row. When this produced no reaction, Rinkel assumed he had misdiagnosed himself.

Many years later, still suffering from chronic health problems, Rinkel decided to eliminate eggs completely from his diet and found that his symptoms receded. But on his sixth eggless day, he took a bite of angel-food cake containing egg, and fainted dead away. This experience led to Rinkel's understanding that some patients who showed symptoms of allergy might be ingesting foods regularly without realizing the foods were causing an allergic response. He coined his discovery *masked allergy*.

Cellular Theory Comes of Age

The cellular theory for the immune system, which had been suggested in the nineteenth century, had to wait until the 1940s for a revival of interest and ultimate discovery. It took more work in the areas of immunodeficiency and autoimmunity before the idea of cell-mediated immunity was completely accepted into the mainstream. Cellular immunology finally came into its own in the 1950s.

As time went on, studies were made of patients who had nonfunctioning or only partially functioning immune systems to protect them against harmful bacteria. This condition is called *deficient immunity* or *immunodeficiency*. Another group studied had an immune system that mistakenly recognized their own tissue (self) as being foreign tissue (nonself), (*auto* meaning "self-immunity" or "immunity against oneself").

In 1967, four years after the death of Carl Prausnitz, the Japanese-American husband and wife team Teruko and Kimishige Ishizaka isolated a reagin part of the serum of a patient who was sensitive to ragweed. Rabbits immunized with this produced antibodies. When the reagin-rich substance was mixed with the antiserum, a new allergy antibody was formed and identified: gamma E globulin, to be renamed immunoglobulin E or IgE at the World Health Organization (WHO) conference in 1968. The Ishizakas not only discovered IgE antibodies, but proved they were identical with the reaginic antibodies identified some 45 years earlier by Prausnitz and Küstner.

Milestones in Allergy Medicine

The following list provides a timeline of important discoveries and contributions in the field of allergy medicine and immunology over the past two centuries:

Year	Name	Contribution
1798	Edward Jenner	Pioneers smallpox vaccination
1862	Ernst Haeckel	Identifies phagocytosis
1877	Paul Erlich	Identifies mast cells
1879	Louis Pasteur	Pioneers vaccinations to immunity against viral diseases
1883	Ilya Metchnikoff	Theorizes that cells are involved in the defense of the body
1891	Robert Koch	Discovers delayed type hypersensitivity
1895	Jules Bordet	Observes complement and antibody activity
1900	Paul Erlich	Theorizes that antibodies are involved in allergic reactions
1902	Charles Richet	Coins the term anaphylaxis to describe the most dangerous allergic reaction
1906	Clemens von Pirquet	Coins the word allergy
1907	Arrhenius, Svante	Coins the term immunochemistry
1910	Sir Henry Dale	Identifies histamine, a body chemical responsible for many allergic reactions
1916	Robert Cook Albert Vander Veer	Demonstrate the role of heredity in allergy sufferers
1921	Carl Prausnitz Heinz Küstner	Discover that components in the blood can reproduce food allergy reactions
1926	Loyd D. Felton and Bailey	Isolates pure antibody preparation

Year	Name	Contribution
1934	John Marrack	Advances the antigen-antibody binding hypothesis
1937	David Bovet	Synthesizes the first antihistamine
1940	Karl Landsteiner Alexander S. Weiner	Identify Rh antigens
1941	Albert Coons	Develops immunofluorescence technique
1942	Karl Landsteiner Merril Chase	Discover the cellular transfer of sensitivity (anaphylaxis)
1948	Astrid Fagraeus	Demonstrates the production of antibodies in plasma B cells
1950	Howard Gershon Koichi S. Kondo	Discover suppressor T cells
1953	J. F. Riley G. B. West	Discover histamine in mast cells
1958	Jean Dausset	Discovers human leukocyte antigens
1959	Rodney Porter	Discovers antibody structure
1964	Anthony Davis	Identifies T and B cell cooperation in immune response
1967	Teruko and Kimishige Ishizaka	Identify IgE, the allergy antibody
1985	Susumu Tonegawa	Identifies immunoglobulin genes
1985	Leroy Hood	Identifies genes for the T cell receptor
1990	NIH team	Advances gene therapy using cultured T cells
2000	FDA	Approves the first anti-IgE drug, rhu-MAb-E25

What We Know About Allergic Reactions Today

Today we know that allergic reactions are the result of an over-reactive immune system, which has the remarkable ability to defend what it recognizes as the body (self) against that which it has been programmed to recognize as an invader or antigen/allergen (nonself). These antigens/allergens can sneak into the body from many directions. They may enter as food, pollen, insect bites, drugs, or bacteria through the skin, the mouth, the nose, the eyes, or any other body orifice.

Introducing the Key Players

The immune system is made up of a number of cells all coming from the family called *white blood cells* (WBCs), which includes so-called *leukocytes* such as macrophage and basophil cells and *lymphocytes* such as T and B cells. This group of cells acts collectively to protect us from invasion of foreign bodies such as bacteria or viruses, by surrounding an invader and engulfing it or eating it, then digesting it with chemicals stored inside the WBCs. In the process, some WBCs release chemicals that cause body temperature to rise, so fever is really a part of the body's defense system.

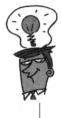

Bet You Didn't Know _____

Lymphocytes such as T cells and B cells originate in stem cells in the bone marrow. Unlike T cells, however, which travel through the circulatory system to the thymus gland where they mature, B cells travel to an area, we think, in the digestive tract, where the environment influences them to grow into adult B cells. When mature, these cells then travel to our lymph glands, where they wait to respond for our protection.

Macrophage cells are the first strong arm to greet the invader—*macro* means "large," and *phage* means "to eat or destroy." These cells form a barrier to the spread of harmful invaders, while alerting the rest of the system to join in the battle against the antigens. More specifically, macrophage cells are in charge of the cell movement of other WBCs that surround foreign materials, and of introducing the antigen they engulf to the T cells, which are charged with identifying the invader. After the introduction has been made—by actually "docking" to the T cell (like a spaceship docks to a space station)—the T cell sends chemical signals to the B cell, which in turn creates a "memory" B cell that stores all available information about the antigen.

Bet You Didn't Know _____

The immune system starts at birth and gradually develops and matures over the first six months of the infant's life and beyond, through a series of exposures to antigens. With each exposure, the immune system gradually builds up a better protective shield in the form of Ig antibodies. IgM and IgG antibodies are formed first, followed by IgE, IgA, and IgD antibodies.

B cells are like manufacturing plants that produce one of five antigen-specific proteins called *immunoglobulin* (Ig). For example, if the invader is a bacteria or virus, then the B cells generate IgG or IgM antibodies to fight infections. To protect tissue in the digestive tract against harmful materials in secretions (such as saliva) and prevent certain proteins from going directly into the bloodstream, B cells produce IgA antibodies. To protect the body against parasitic infections, B cells manufacture IgE antibodies, which are also prominent in allergic reactions. (To date, scientists can only theorize as to the purpose of IgD, which rounds out the body's immunoglobulin collection).

Each immunoglobulin is programmed to search out an antigen in its original form. The next time the antigen comes into circulation, this series of events repeats itself, with the proviso that now the "memory" B cell divides itself many times, each time producing the appropriate immunoglobulin proteins. The immunoglobulin is then sent on its way to search out and destroy any foreign substance that is *exactly* the same as identified in the memory B cell. This process is generally referred to as *specificity*.

Med Meaning _____

Specificity refers to the process when an individual immunoglobulin is programmed to search out an antigen in its original form, which is crucial for the immune system to react to an antigen to which it has been sensitized. Change the molecular structure of the antigen slightly—raw carrots the first time, cooked carrots the next—and the system may let it go on by without a reaction.

When Things Get Ugly

In IgE-mediated immune system reactions—those triggered by IgE antibodies—B cells produce the IgE antibodies in response to a chemical signal produced by the aforementioned T cells. These IgE antibodies then attach to two other important players in an allergic reaction—mast cells in lining tissue and basophils in blood. The next time the allergen enters the body again, its protein attaches to the waiting IgE antibodies, which in turn triggers the mast cells and basophils to fall apart or degranulate. In this process, the cells release preformed mediators such as histamine and other chemicals that travel through the bloodstream to the area that causes the familiar allergic symptoms, such as swelling, itching, hives, or sneezing. In the lungs, these chemicals can cause muscle spasms which in turn narrows the breathing passages, making it more difficult to breath.

Timely Tip _____

Taking antihistamines daily during a known allergy season will work better for the patient than taking them only after symptoms occur. Antihistamines are more effective before the mast cell is exposed to antigens and releases its stored-up histamine.

The following figure illustrates the basic steps that lead to an allergic reaction.

The allergic process: from sensitization to reaction.

Initial Exposure

Allergen

White blood cell

Antibodies

Mast cell

Basophil

1. First contact with allergen causes white blood cells to produce IgE antibodies

2. The IgE antibodies attach to mast cells in tissue lining and basophils in blood

Re-exposure

Mediators ➞

3. When the same allergen enters the body again, its proteins attach to the waiting IgE antibodies

4. IgE antibodies trigger the mast cells and basophils to degranulate and release chemicals such as histamine that are responsible for allergic distress

---

Typecasting Immune System Reactions

Immune system reactions can occur within minutes after exposure to the offending allergen, and can last up to three days, if tissue swelling is involved. Other reactions may not occur until hours or days after exposure to the allergen. To help explain the different types of immune system responses, the scientific community distinguishes four types of immune system reactions:

- ◆ Type I reactions, also know as immediate onset, IgE-mediated, or atopic reactions, develop in stages. The first encounter with an antigen sensitizes and stimulates B cells to produce IgE specific to the intruding allergen. An example of this type of reaction is a food allergy.

- ◆ Type II reactions, also known as antibody-mediated cytotoxic histamine, involve IgG antibodies and are a delayed reaction. An example is the Rh Factor in newborns.

- ◆ Type III, or immune complex reactions, involve antigen complexes that are too large to be engulfed and destroyed by WBCs, and are deposited in tissue where they simulate destructive inflammation. An example of this type of reaction is inflammation of the kidney, called *nephritis*.

- ◆ Type IV reactions, also known as delayed hypersensitivity, don't show symptoms until 24 or more hours after exposure to the allergen. A good example is a poison ivy reaction.

Treatment for each of these conditions varies with the severity of the reaction and the general medical condition of the patient. This is especially true if the patient has other medical problems which may prohibit one medication or another.

The origins of the immune system process can be traced back to the beginning of life, in the form of single-celled organisms such as paramecium or amoeba. These microscopic life-forms engulfed an enemy by surrounding it, chemically digesting it, and then excreting it. Over many generations, while life developed into more complex multiple-cell organisms, the process of tackling invaders, however, has remained the same as for a single-celled organism, with the proviso that the human immune system has evolved into a network of cells specializing in definite functions.

The Least You Need to Know

- Since ancient times, people have observed that the consumption of harmless substances can create health problems in some people.

- The word allergy was coined in the beginning of the twentieth century.

- The antibody involved in food allergies was fully isolated and proved in the 1960s.

- Allergic reactions are the result of the immune system overreacting to harmless substances.

The Many Faces and Places of Food Allergies

In This Chapter

- Defining adverse food reactions
- Identifying symptoms of a true food allergy
- Understanding anaphylaxis
- Gauging the chances of outgrowing a food allergy

Food allergies can show up in many ways. They can affect any and all of the systems of the body, and can appear as a variety of different symptoms. This chapter helps you identify true food allergies and their symptoms. To do this you must have a clear picture of what constitutes a nonallergic, food intolerance type of reaction.

Defining Adverse Reactions to Food

The reported incidence of food allergy around the world is divergent. Figures range from 2 percent all the way to 15 percent. This disagreement is probably due to the fact that different criteria are being used and food allergy is being defined in different ways.

According to the National Institutes of Health (NIH) and the American Academy of Allergy, Asthma, and Clinical Immunology, problems with food should be referred to as "adverse food reactions." However, this is a generic classification for any unusual or harmful reaction after the ingestion of food, and does not specify whether the reaction is a *true food allergy* or simply a food intolerance. In general, most scientists agree that a true allergic reaction to food can be defined as an inappropriate immune system response that causes symptoms in some allergy-prone people. Food intolerance, by contrast, is the result of nonimmunologic mechanisms. (For more details on food intolerance see Chapter 4.)

Med Meaning

True food allergy occurs through factors in the lining of the gastrointestinal tract, and usually involves IgE-mediated reactions to a specific food. It also involves the immunoglobulin attacking a food antigen already attached to certain cells in the bloodstream.

Confusing Variables

Gauging the frequency of true food allergies is also made worse by immune factors that are changing within the gastrointestinal tract—from very little protection to full protection, based on the age of the patient. The body's systems are constantly changing, as are the body's reactions.

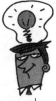

Bet You Didn't Know

Most practicing allergists feel that allergic reactions to food occur in about 2 percent of the general population.

A person must have normal levels of IgA antibodies to block foods from causing allergies. These IgA antibodies can be found in the normal secretions of the stomach lining. However, at birth, when the protective immune system is still immature, the IgA level is zero, so the body must start producing its own IgA antibodies. On average, it takes about four months or more to produce enough IgA antibodies to reach near adult levels.

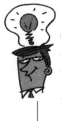

Bet You Didn't Know

Oral tolerance is a protective happening that usually occurs early in life. The immune system does not react to intact protein entering the circulation. This is not well understood, but it is thought that the cells of the immune system develop a tolerance to intact nutrient proteins. This occurs in the first few weeks when the newborn needs all the nutrient protein it can get.

Furthermore, a baby's basic acid level is very low at birth, and does not reach adult levels until one month of age. Proteolytic enzymes, which are necessary to break down protein, do not reach adult activity level until two years of age. In other words, infants have minimal ways to stop large protein molecules—the form before digestion—from crossing the barrier into the circulation. When large protein molecules appear, the immune system recognizes them as foreign and dangerous and reacts accordingly. In short, when you look at a child's development of the immune system in the digestive tract it presents a different picture with the passage of time. A snapshot taken at different times in the stage of the developing gastrointestinal tract provides a different impression of frequency of food allergies.

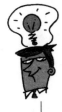

Bet You Didn't Know

Infantile colic is not well defined, and involves intermittent fussiness plus agonized crying, drawing up of the legs, distention of the abdomen, and excessive gas. Colic starts in the first two to four weeks of life and lasts into the third or fourth month of life. There is no one known cause, but recent studies with bottle-fed and breast-fed infants suggest the condition is related to food allergies in about 10 percent of those infants studied.

Inside the Stomach Immune System

The human body has a police system called *gut-associated lymphoid tissue* (*GALT*) to protect it from potential bacterial invaders. This police force is composed of lymphocyte white blood cells, which are spread out in at least three locations, one of which is called *lamina propria lymphocytes*. Scattered in one layer of the digestive tract, a majority of these cells are B cells that produce IgA.

When certain foreign substances that contain protein antigens come into play, a cell called the *microfold* or *M cell* appears and engulfs the protein. M-cells report to the *macrophage cells* or large eating cells (see Chapter 2). The macrophages go directly to the T cells. These T cells then send chemical signals to B cells, which in turn divide themselves repeatedly to produce IgA-secreting cells.

These same B cells also produce a joining piece called a *J-chain*, which holds together two molecules of IgA, which in this form is called *S-IgA*. When this new, larger molecule gets into the secretions of the digestive tract it hooks on to the invading bacteria, and creates an even larger molecule. Because only the smallest molecules can get through the opening in the digestive tract into the bloodstream, this larger molecule cannot escape into the bloodstream to hide and do harm and is trapped instead in the digestive tract, where it is engulfed and destroyed by white blood cells.

continues

continued

One of the prime tasks IgA performs is protecting us against foreign substances such as bacteria, viruses, and undigested food proteins invading the body. The IgA is in the secretions of the body such as in the intestinal tract. Not having enough IgA means we can have more infections than usual. Commonly, this happens in the sinuses and middle ear, but also in the intestinal tract. It's the IgA that prevents all protein bacteria and food protein from getting into the bloodstream. In infancy, too little IgA allows some food protein into circulation before it is digested or broken down. Introducing solid food before four months of age means that large protein molecules are coming into the digestive tract before the infant has enough S-IgA to stop it from going into the circulation. The body recognizes this as something foreign, and sets up an allergic response the next time that particular substance is taken in. One of the first steps in a food allergy in infancy could be that the infant has not produced enough IgA as yet. Breast-feeding provides easily digested protein, as well as some S-IgA from the mother's milk to help protect against future food allergies. (For more information on breast-feeding see Chapter 10.)

Gutsy Moves

The speed at which food proteins can penetrate the gut walls depends on various conditions, not the least on whether the patient has an empty stomach. In one historical experiment mentioned in Chapter 2, a doctor took serum from a patient known to be fish and egg allergic. He put this serum under the skin of a nonegg- and nonfish-allergic patient. Twenty-four hours later, he fed this patient fish, and that patient developed a red swollen area where the injection had been given. This shows that the patient had been sensitized within 24 hours or less.

Today, we can use similar studies in safer ways, by measuring the specific IgE levels in known allergic patients. From these studies, it has been shown that peanuts are absorbed orally in 24.3 minutes; from the duodenum in 18.6 minutes; and from the rectum in 18.7 minutes. Food is absorbed faster from the small intestine, colon, and rectum, and slower from the esophagus and stomach. The importance of all this is to appreciate how quickly a food reaction can possibly occur after eating the food.

Bet You Didn't Know

Some medications are given in suppository form, especially if the patient cannot retain anything in the stomach due to vomiting. Because the rectum has a large amount of blood vessels, medications applied here are absorbed very quickly into the circulation. This same situation exists under the tongue, in the nose, and in the eye sac.

Factors that decrease the rate of absorption of food antigens are many, including increased stomach acid, other food in the gut, and the ingestion of kaolin, which is found in Kaopectate. Factors that increase the rate of absorption are decreased stomach acidity and alcohol. Medication is absorbed more quickly when taken on an empty stomach, and requires a longer time to work after a large meal.

Down Another Pipeline

Food travels from your mouth down the esophagus into the gastrointestinal tract. Some researchers argue that some of the food actually can react with IgE and mast cells in the throat to cause allergic reactions in the nose, throat, and eyes.

Other researchers maintain that food molecules go into the circulation and to the end organ within minutes. Why does the antigen go to one area before another? Why to one area and not another? This is still a mystery. What is known is that food allergies causing problems only in the respiratory tract (lungs, nose, and sinuses) are not as common as food allergies causing problems in the skin or gastrointestinal tract.

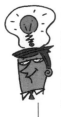

Bet You Didn't Know

Symptoms such as runny or stuffy nose and/or sneezing are often signs of rhinitis. Usually food allergies involve the gastrointestinal tract and skin. They can also cause symptoms in the respiratory tract, such as the nose. The age-old question of "Is it related to ear infection?" has not been answered. However, it seems that when allergies are controlled, ear infections tend to decrease in some people.

The Elephant on Your Chest

In a real food allergy reaction in the breathing areas, you might have molecules of food antigen coming into the area through the blood vessels. The watchdog IgE antibodies, attached to mast cells or basophil white blood cells, hook up to the food antigen. The resulting allergic process (described in detail in Chapter 2) starts, with the result that blood vessels in the area dilate, muscles contract around the breathing tubes, and great amounts of mucous are produced. The patient commonly complains of an elephant sitting on his chest, because he cannot expand the chest to take in air. The muscles around the breathing tubes contract, so the airway is narrowed and blocked by the extra mucous.

That Itchy Mouth of Yours

Another set of symptoms that can occur in food-allergic people is called the *oral allergy syndrome*. In this case, symptoms in the mouth and throat occur following eating certain foods, commonly after eating fresh fruit and vegetables, but symptoms do not go on to cause generalized allergic reactions throughout the body. The reaction in patients allergic to ragweed appear when eating fresh melon, especially watermelon, cantaloupe, and honeydew, as well as bananas. Patients allergic to birch tree pollen may have problems with fresh apples and hazelnuts. Latex-sensitive patients commonly complain about reactions to kiwi, banana, and avocado, among other foods. Symptoms— itching in the mouth, swelling of the lips, tongue, roof of the mouth, and throat— occur when eating the specific food. There are reports of blisters on the lining of the mouth and even tightening of the throat.

The Dreaded "A" Word—Anaphylaxis

Anaphylaxis is the most severe of the allergic reactions. A good description of anaphylaxis is quick onset, with severe, sometimes fatal, reactions. This is usually related directly, and within a very short time, to the exposure of a single agent (food, medication, insect bites) to which the patient has been sensitized through a previous exposure. The list of causes are many, and include antibiotics such as penicillin, aspirin, allergen extracts used for allergy desensitization, radiopaque dyes used in x-ray studies; venoms such as honeybee, wasp, hornet, or yellow jacket; blood products such as whole blood or gammaglobulin; and foods, especially egg whites, cow's milk, shellfish, tree nuts, and peanuts. Latex products can also cause this distress in a latex-sensitive person.

> **Med Meaning**
>
> **Anaphylaxis** is a generalized allergic reaction that involves many systems of the body, including the heart, lungs, kidneys, and blood vessels. Capillaries dilate and muscles contract, which may result in a drop in blood pressure, difficulty breathing, slowing or stopping of the heart, and possible kidney shutdown.

The Skinny on Anaphylaxis

A true anaphylactic reaction occurs through the IgE portion of the immune system. The antigen or allergen cause of the reaction will crosslink with the IgE antibodies on the surface of mast cells and basophils. These cells then release the mediating chemicals, which create changes in the blood vessels and bring other white blood cells into the area. These in turn release more chemicals in other parts of the body. The chance of this happening is more frequent in someone with allergies.

A reaction can occur with varying amounts of severity. The mildest form would be a local reaction such as hives, followed by swelling. The reaction can be very strong, but is rarely fatal. A more severe form of reaction would involve many areas of the body, including the lungs, heart, gastrointestinal tract, and skin.

The symptoms of this systemic, generalized allergic reaction can start with mild conditions of skin tingling or itching, moving on to a feeling of warmth. Some people will notice a fullness in the mouth and throat, along with congestion in the nose and swelling around the eyes. Eye tearing and sneezing can also occur. The start of these symptoms is usually within the first 30 minutes after exposure, but can progress gradually over a two-hour period. In the worst-case scenario, a sufferer can go into anaphylactic shock, losing consciousness due to choking or a drop in blood pressure. People with food allergies who also suffer from asthma are believed to be at a higher risk for developing an anaphylactic reaction. Food-induced anaphylaxis is said to cause about 30,000 trips to the emergency room and between 150 to 200 deaths each year in the United States.

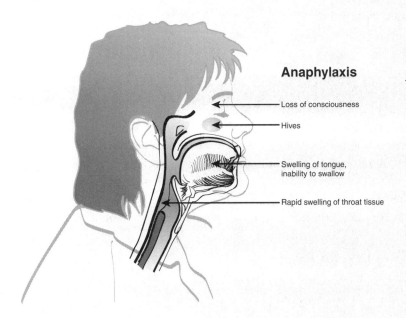

Anaphylaxis

— Loss of consciousness

— Hives

— Swelling of tongue, inability to swallow

— Rapid swelling of throat tissue

This figure shows the effects of anaphylaxis, a dangerous condition that can happen to food allergy sufferers, causing unconsciousness or even death.

Immediate treatment with appropriate safe medication can reverse or stop the chain of events. This series of allergic symptoms can progress to spasm and swelling in the lungs, with the person becoming short of breath, coughing, and wheezing. Skin flushing is common, as is itching, nausea, vomiting, and a sense of anxiety. The most serious symptoms can progress to severe spasm of the lungs, swelling in the throat, hoarseness, and difficulty breathing. Other systems of the body become involved, including the urinary system with cramping of the bladder, the central nervous system causing seizures, and finally the heart can collapse, with a drop in blood pressure. These symptoms can occur again in the next 8 to 12 hours.

Deadly Enemies

Typical symptoms of anaphylaxis include the following:
- ◆ Swelling of the throat, lips, or tongue
- ◆ Difficulty breathing or swallowing
- ◆ Metallic taste or itching in the mouth
- ◆ Flushing, itching, redness of the skin (hives)
- ◆ Nausea
- ◆ Increased heart rate
- ◆ Lowered blood pressure
- ◆ Sudden feeling of weakness
- ◆ Anxiety or an overwhelming sense of doom
- ◆ Collapse and loss of consciousness

Treatment with self-injectable epinephrine is important in the first stages of the reaction. The patient or surrogate can be trained to do this. The epinephrine will usually help to stop or reverse the life-threatening events. Once again, a physician should determine what type of medication the patient should have available. This decision depends on other medical problems such as heart or blood pressure problems and what medications the patient may be taking. If the reaction is severe, the patient should be cared for in an emergency room for respiratory support and treatment of shock.

So You Thought Exercise Was All Good

There is another reaction to foods that is similar to anaphylaxis and is called *anaphylactoid reaction*. This means anaphylactic-like reaction. This reaction is similar to anaphylaxis, but is not caused by the antigen/allergen/IgE pathway in the immune system. It works through another, parallel immune system in the body called the *complement system*. In this case, the trigger reacts on the complement directly to release the mediators that then cause the problem. An example of this is a situation called *food-dependent, exercise-induced anaphylaxis (F-EIA)*. Some allergic people will have severe anaphylactoid reactions when exercising after eating certain foods. There is no one food that is generally responsible, but the culprit is usually one specific food unique to that patient. The reaction can occur

Skulls and Bones

Although virtually any food can trigger anaphylaxis, in most cases the culprits causing this condition are the same 8 major offending foods that cause 80 to 90 percent of the less harmful allergic reactions: peanuts, tree nuts, shellfish, milk, eggs, and fish. Anaphylaxis is an extremely severe form of an allergic reaction.

up to two hours after eating the offending food, followed by exercise, including vigorous dancing. In some cases a specific food is noted, while in other cases it can be any meal preceding the exercise.

Worst of the Worst

For people who suffer from food allergies, the worst allergic reactions occur to peanuts, tree nuts, and shellfish. The most sudden reactions, or ones that cause generalized, serious anaphylaxis, are those foods that the person does not routinely eat—usually because they know they are allergic to that food.

When patients have an anaphylactic reaction to food, usually one or more of these factors is found in the history of the patient:

- The patient has unknowingly eaten the offending food.
- The patient has bronchial asthma.
- The patient has a history of previous reactions.

All reactions are immediate, and the afflicted patient is usually helped dramatically with epinephrine (also called adrenaline).

It has been advised that people with known food allergies, especially those with a history of severe generalized reactions, should have a source of epinephrine immediately available. In the case of children, it is carried by the parents. While at school, it should be with the school nurse, teacher, or school administration. There are different kinds available, depending on the age of the patient, and so on. The choice should be determined by the patient's doctor. These recommendations come from the American Academy and the College of Allergy, as well as other knowledgeable sources.

CAUTION

Skulls and Bones

One of the biggest problems those with food allergies face is verifying whether a forbidden ingredient is contained in a particular food. Deaths have occurred because people were unaware the food they ate contained a substance to which they were allergic. In adults the most common foods that cause food allergies are fish, shellfish, tree nuts, wheat, corn, and peanuts, which are the most likely to cause anaphylactic shock. In children the foods include eggs, cow's milk, tree nuts, and peanuts. Foods touching the skin and causing problems are usually meat and dairy products, fish, raw vegetables, and fruits. Symptoms caused by these foods are usually of short duration, and appear as chronic skin problems no more than 1 to 2 percent of the time.

The most common areas of the body to be affected are the gastrointestinal tract and the skin. In the case of the gastrointestinal tract, the mediators involved include histamine, which will cause swelling, cramping, pain, nausea, vomiting, and diarrhea as the body tries to rid itself of the offending food. With skin symptoms, there can be severe itching, flushing, and welts. Some parts of the body, such as the face, hands, feet, and genital area, may have marked swelling. Here the histamine causes the blood vessels to release fluid into the tissues, which results in swelling. Patients with atopic dermatitis may have increased problems if they are allergic to certain foods—eggs, cow's milk, peanuts, or fish being the most prominent.

Atopic dermatitis, also known as eczema, is a name given to itching with a rash of allergic cause. An Italian physician named Paolo Bagellardo first described atopic dermatitis in a pediatric medical book titled *Libellus de Aegretudinibus Infantium*. In 1800, Bessner gave an understandable description and called it *atopic* (allergic) *dermatitis* (skin inflammation). He noted that the condition ran in families or was hereditary, and was usually associated with allergic rhinitis and bronchial asthma. The name atopic dermatitis emphasizes that this form is somehow related to being allergic.

All the evidence pointing to atopic dermatitis being a form of allergy is indirect but convincing. First, about 75 percent of patients with atopic dermatitis have increased amounts of IgE specific for food. Elimination of specific foods from the diet for one year can result in a decrease of eczema symptoms. Usually the cause of the allergic reaction is a specific food in a group of foods, not all the foods in a food group. An example is that peanuts are in the legume group, with peas, beans, and soy being other members of the group. However, there is a crossover in some foods—90 percent of people allergic to cow's milk are also allergic to goat's milk; 40 percent of people allergic to beef will react to lamb.

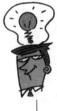

Bet You Didn't Know

The skin is a frequent target or end organ for food allergy reactions. The allergy has many forms, but most commonly comes out as hives or tissue swelling.

Adios, Allergy?

Routinely eaten foods that cause allergies result in symptoms in areas of chronic problems such as the skin with eczema or the lungs with asthma. Patients showing these symptoms are usually younger—anywhere from infancy to early childhood. A person with a combination of atopic dermatitis plus food allergies can be at risk for having respiratory problems. A patient with chronic or difficult-to-control asthma in some cases also has food allergies.

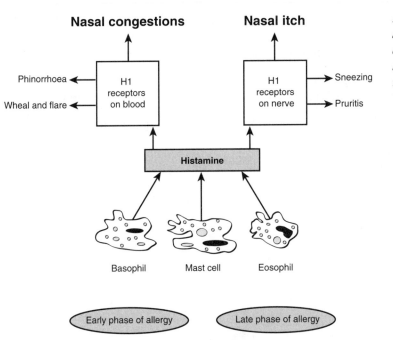

Food allergies frequently attack the respiratory system, causing all varieties of problems, from simple nasal itch to severe asthma.

So does this go on forever? The natural history is that one third of patients with atopic dermatitis and food allergies will outgrow the problem. About 20 percent of children with eczema have food allergies. The chance of the food allergy disappearing depends on three things:

- ◆ The foods involved. For example, if the allergy is to soy, wheat, milk, or eggs, it can disappear, while if the allergy is to peanuts, tree nuts, fish, or shellfish, it probably will not disappear.

- ◆ How high the IgE level is to an individual food.

- ◆ The degree to which the patient sticks to an elimination or avoidance diet (see Chapter 8 for details on elimination diets).

Some researchers advise to sample with known allergic foods every one to three years in very small amounts. However, this is dangerous, even life-threatening, to do with peanuts, tree nuts, or shellfish. The safest approach would be to consult your physician before trying this. It would be safer to do this where there is emergency help available in case of a severe reaction. The best approach with this group of foods, or even other foods that have caused severe reactions in the past, is to eliminate them completely from the diet and do not risk a challenge at any time. There are case reports where patients, challenged in an emergency room setting with adrenaline and life support equipment readily available, have not responded to treatment and have died.

The Least You Need to Know

♦ A true food allergy involves the immune system and immunoglobulin proteins.

♦ Food antigens can travel through the bloodstream to end organs such as the lungs, skin, and upper respiratory system as well as the digestive system.

♦ Most of the food-allergic reaction is immediate and short, and it can be life-threatening.

♦ Awareness of food content is important to avoid exposure whenever possible.

Part 2

Bring on the Food

Let's face it, food causes one sort of problem or another for just about everybody at some time. Whether you are or aren't allergic to a particular food, it's important you learn the various corners from which foods can attack: foods that contain histamine, foods with toxic agents, contaminated food—we'll sort out the underlying villains to help identify the real cause of your food-related problem.

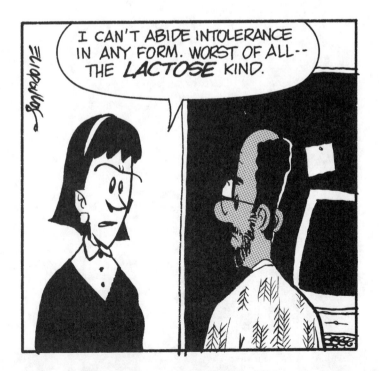

Chapter 4

Food as a Troublemaker

In This Chapter

- Take a look at food problems that are not food allergies
- Learn about the toxic agents in food
- Know what the pharmacologic agents in food are
- Find out about metabolic reactions and food

Of all people who have problems with food, it is estimated by practicing allergists that only about 2 percent suffer from true food allergies, while the remaining 98 percent have nonallergic reactions to food. These reactions might be triggered by natural chemicals within the food, or contamination of the food with any number of substances. The real importance, then, is sorting out the underlying causes, because contaminants can not only elicit immediate symptoms that might mimic those of a true food allergy, but may cause permanent, serious damage to other organs in the body. This chapter provides an overview of food-related problems that have nothing to do with food allergies.

Defining Food Intolerance

The term *food intolerance* is used in different ways by different physicians. One meaning is "an abnormal response by the body to a food or food additive that has been eaten." This reaction is not through the body's immunologic system (as is the case in a true food allergy), but through contaminants in the foods or chemical parts in certain foods.

These factors include toxic contaminants such as bacteria that cause a chemical reaction in fish, or actual toxins in the fish themselves. Another factor could be traced to the pharmacologic properties of the food, such as reactions to caffeine in coffee or tyramine in aged cheese.

Med Meaning

Idiosyncrasy comes from two words, *idios*, meaning "one's own," plus *synkrasis*, meaning "a mixing together." Health professionals use the word to mean an abnormal reaction to a drug or a chemical, or an opposite response.

A third type of food intolerance can be the result of characteristics within the person's own body or system. Examples of this are lactose deficiency, or an opposite reaction to chemicals called *idiosyncratic* response. Here, for example, a person usually gets sleepy after taking an antihistamine like Benadryl. The opposite reaction is when one becomes stimulated, anxious, or unable to sleep after taking this medication.

Symptoms Commonly Blamed on Food Allergy

The following table provides an overview of symptoms that are commonly blamed on food allergies and the type of food that causes them.

Symptoms	Foods/Possible Causes
Abdominal pain and cramps	High-fiber foods, lactose intolerance, vitamins, diet supplements
Rectal gas and belching	Cabbage, cucumbers, beans, berries, lactose intolerance, carbonated drinks, high-fat diet
Frequent bowel movements	Fruit, foods with high sugar content, large quantity of juice, high-fiber foods
Frequent urinations	Large quantities of fluids, bladder infection
Runny nose	Spicy food, large quantities of food
Itching, welts, and swelling	Licorice, foods with high salt content, strawberries
Fast heartbeat, nervousness, and insomnia	Foods with caffeine

What's in That Thing Called Food?

Some foods naturally contain a wide variety of active chemicals that can create symptoms such as headaches, itching, stuffy nose, or sneezing.

One chemical group is called *vasoactive amines*. Included in this group is histamine, a chemical agent released in IgE-mediated allergic reactions to food (see Chapter 2 for details). Bacteria that break down amino acids produce these vasoactive amines. Examples include tyramine in cheese, histamine in contaminated tuna, and phenylethylamine in chocolate. Some amines are found naturally in bananas, tomatoes, plums, pineapples, avocados, oranges, and red wine. These amines can cause headaches, and can also interact with some medications.

Another group of foods contains agents that can cause psychological or neurological problems. Some are stimulants—LSD, myristin in nutmeg, opiate in peyote, pyridines in nicotine, tetrahydrocannabinols in hemp, and caffeine or theobromine in coffee, tea, cola, chocolate, and cocoa. Patients have reported symptoms such as nervousness, anxiety, and abdominal pain from taking in these substances. With some of these stimulants, such as caffeine and nicotine, it depends on the amount used.

Bet You Didn't Know

There are 55 mg of caffeine in 12 ounces of cola; 150 mg of caffeine in one cup of coffee; and 200 mg of theobromine in a 4-ounce chocolate bar.

Natural Poisons

Another example of food intolerance is known as *anaphylactoid reaction*, which mimics the symptoms of an anaphylactic reaction to food, but may in reality be a reaction to contaminated food or food additives that cause allergylike symptoms.

Scombroid fish, such as tuna, mackerel, and mahi mahi, can be involved in this type of poisoning. These fish must be refrigerated at proper low temperatures immediately after being caught. The fish can be contaminated with bacteria called *Proteus morganii* or *Klebsiella pneumoniae*. If allowed to grow in the fish, the bacteria can react on natural *histadine* found in the fish tissue. The bacteria break down the histadine to histamine.

The histamine produced as a result of this process reaches very high concentrations in the fish when it is prepared and eaten. This literally becomes histamine poisoning. The symptoms are erythema or flushing, itchy eyes, headache, and gastrointestinal upset.

Persons taking the medicine INH (isoniazid) are very susceptible to this type of histamine. INH is used for patients exposed to tuberculosis. Diagnosis of histamine poisoning is made on the basis of allergylike symptoms and finding the food to have very high levels of histamine. The symptoms are easily reversible.

CAUTION

Skulls and Bones _____

Avoid eating spoiled tuna, mackerel, mahi mahi, or any fish kept at high storage temperatures. Contaminated fish has a sharp, peppery, metallic taste.

Other examples of food that can have adverse changes by contamination are bacteria in well-ripened cheese (especially Swiss cheese), and unrefrigerated salami-like sausages. This has also been reported to occur with sauerkraut, red wine, and champagne, and less commonly in white wine and beer. (White wine and beer have lower amounts of histamine.)

Histamine Straight Up

There is a long list of other foods that normally contain histamine, which can cause allergylike symptoms to occur. These include some canned fish, sauerkraut, mixed alcoholic drinks, bananas, ketchup, soy sauce, spinach, strawberries, and yeast.

The symptoms of histamine intoxication are nausea, diarrhea, skin rashes, flushing, and headaches. Normally the liver removes histamine in about twelve hours, unless the patient has cirrhosis, which decreases liver function.

Foods That Can Poison

Many common foods contain toxins, but in very low concentrations, so that reactions are infrequent. Real problems show up when the foods are eaten in very large amounts or prepared in unusual ways. Human poisoning can occur in four different ways:

- Foods that are known to be unsafe.
- Food contaminants eaten in large quantities that will cause problems.
- Foods eaten in large quantities that will cause problems.
- Foods that affect a select group of people.

Foods Known to Be Unsafe

Persons experimenting with hallucinogenic plants, trying wilderness survival techniques, or eating food harvested in their natural state are at risk. Problems occur when experimenting with Psilocybe or Amanita mushrooms, or when eating them by mistake. A third possibility for a problem would be eating a large quantity of these mushrooms. All of these can lead to toxicity.

There are other poisonous plants that are grown in gardens. An example includes foxglove—known to most as *digitalis purpurea*—which contains digitoxin. Eating this plant can cause severe, if not fatal, heart problems. Another plant called *groundsel* contains a poison called *pyrrolizide alkaloid*.

Some animals are unsafe to eat. The puffer fish, a Japanese delicacy, and some types of salamander are poisonous if eaten.

Some foods have dangerous levels of toxins, but only in special situations. Green potatoes have high levels of glycoalkaloids. Certain lima bean varieties have high cyanogenic glycosides. There are poisonous chemicals in raw, uncooked red beans which will cause severe gastrointestinal problems. Raw cottonseed has toxic fractions within it.

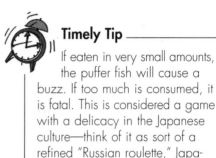

Timely Tip

If eaten in very small amounts, the puffer fish will cause a buzz. If too much is consumed, it is fatal. This is considered a game with a delicacy in the Japanese culture—think of it as sort of a refined "Russian roulette," Japanese style.

To the rescue are scientists who are removing toxic fractions from cottonseed so that it can be used safely in animal and human foods. Nontoxic varieties of lima beans have also been developed.

Unsafe if Eaten in Large Quantities—Part I

Some foods contain toxins but are not harmful unless eaten in very large amounts. Foods in this category are plant products, including laetrile. (Remember the so-called miracle cure for cancer? Desperate people were rushing to Mexico to purchase the "magic apricot pit.") People would not naturally be exposed to this.

Laetrile contains cynogenic glycosides that react with stomach acid to form hydrogen cyanide—which is a gas used to execute some criminals given the death sentence.

Other food sources of poisons can come from food not thoroughly cooked, especially when the food in question is consumed in large quantities. Examples include lima beans, cassava root, sorghum, bitter almond, and apricot or peach pits. Cases have also been reported with sweet potatoes, yams, bamboo, maize, and chickpeas. Very, very large amounts of these foods can be fatal. Fad diets that call for "eat nothing but" a particular food, like only grapefruit or apricot or lima beans, for instance, would fall into this category as well. On the other hand, frequently eating small amounts of some of these foods could create low cyanide levels in the blood, which, in turn, could result in loss of balance when walking, or loss of sight.

Tomatoes contain numerous chemicals. In the middle ages, tomatoes were considered a poisonous plant and were avoided. Then someone discovered how great the tomato is on a BLT or hamburger.

Timely Tip _____

To avoid problems, thoroughly cook your food, and avoid eating excessive quantities of potentially dangerous foods at one time. Using moderation is always the best policy.

Here is a list of chemicals in the tomato: Acetaldehyde, ethanol, endosulfan, galactose, histamine, l-glutamic acid methanol (this could start a fire or an engine), red spider mite, serotonin, sodium salicylate, and tryptamine. Each and all of these chemicals can cause symptoms in very large amounts, regardless of the source, whether in tomatoes or other foods.

Unsafe if Eaten in Large Quantities—Part II

Some foods are not poisonous, but eating large amounts can cause side effects in certain parts of the body. For example, so-called goitrogenic compounds, which can be found in any member of the cabbage family, turnips, soybeans, watercress, radishes, rapeseed, and mustard, are chemicals that cause thyroid gland enlargement. Eating iodine will reverse adverse reactions. An easy way to accomplish this is to use iodized table salt.

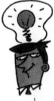

Bet You Didn't Know _____

Thyroid means "resembling a shield." The Greek word is *thyreos,* which means "an oblong shield," plus *eidos,* which means "form" (remember the "Platonic eidos" in Plato's *The Republic?*). The thyroid gland is found in the neck.

Legumes such as peas and beans must be thoroughly cooked, because some will contain chemicals called *hemaglutinins.* These can cause red blood cells to stick together, resulting in blood clots forming in the blood vessels.

Licorice contains a chemical called *glycyrrhizic acid.* In large quantities, this causes sodium retention that, in turn, leads to high blood pressure and possibly enlargement of the heart.

Mushrooms, on the other hand, are high in fiber and have no calories. This is great on a weight loss diet. However, there are some warnings. Some wild mushrooms can cause stomach upset, but the chances of this happening decreases if the mushrooms are thoroughly cooked. Think about the mushroom dilemma when you see raw mushrooms at a salad bar, especially if the owners of the food establishment have picked their own.

Coprinus species mushrooms contain antabuse-type chemicals, which make a person sick if they drink alcohol along with eating the mushroom. Next time you go to a cocktail party, maybe you'll want to look at the canape tray with a jaundiced eye.

Would you believe that large amounts of pepper can cause stomach pain, and that large amounts of nutmeg can lead to psychological problems and liver damage?

An interesting aside: Do you know why your mother told you that when you make a rhubarb pie, to use only the stalk, not the leaves? The reason is that the leaves contain oxalate and anthraquinone glycosides. These can cause intestinal problems or even death.

> **Skulls and Bones**
>
> Coprinus species mushrooms are usually found during autumn in urban regions and along roadsides throughout the United States. One cap of another poisonous mushroom, the Amanita species, can cause death. Amanitas are found in the woods, examples being the Death Cup and the Fly Amanita. Don't be tempted. Be wise. Eat commercially grown mushrooms.

Here's one for you Eskimos. Vitamin A is found in polar bear and chicken liver. Very high doses of Vitamin A can cause toxicity, with vomiting and increased intracranial pressure.

Vitamin D toxicity causes appetite loss, nausea, vomiting, diarrhea, headaches, increased thirst and increased frequency of urination, weight loss, fever, pallor, and/or constipation. Too much of a good thing? Yes; everything in moderation.

Apropos: Too much food or too great a volume of food alone will cause problems. Foods like cucumbers, beans, and berries cause burping, rectal gas, or diarrhea. This will stop by itself, and at worst is annoying and embarrassing.

Foods That Affect but a Few People

Some people are born with or develop a problem due to the lack of certain enzymes needed to break down or digest certain foods. A common example is lactose intolerance. With this condition, a person has small amounts or no lactase enzymes, which are needed to break down lactose, the sugar in milk. Inability to digest the sugar causes bloating, cramps, pain, and, in some people, constipation or diarrhea. Other examples are Phenylketoneuria or PKU and Favism. In each case, the person cannot digest phenylalanine in certain foods with sugar substitutes. In Favism, they cannot eat Vicia fava beans found in Italy.

Food-Related Problems Caused by Medical Conditions

The following list provides an overview of medical conditions that can result in food-related problems:

- ◆ **Favism.** The cause is a phosphate dehydrogenase deficiency. The problem occurs when there is exposure to the Vicia fava beans or pollen from the plant.
- ◆ **Phenylketoneuria (PKU).** The cause is deficiency of phenylalanine hydroxylase. The problem occurs when a person eats foods that contain phenylalanine (commonly found in some artificial sweeteners).
- ◆ **Lactose Intolerance.** The cause is a deficiency of the enzyme lactase, which is needed to break down milk sugars.

Beware of Raw Deals

Food poisoning can occur from a variety of contaminants. These can include algae, bacteria, and the toxic products that they produce. Other less common contaminants are viruses, parasites, rickettsiae, and fungi.

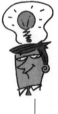

Bet You Didn't Know

Botox, which is used as a fashionable cosmetic treatment to slow down the natural effects of aging, is derived from botulism toxin.

In addition, problems can result from contaminants with environmental pollutants or even inappropriate use of agricultural chemicals. Toxins or chemical contamination act very quickly, within minutes to several hours after ingestion, whereas infection from contaminated food takes eight hours to several days after eating the food for symptoms to occur. Examples include wheat infestation, shellfish infestation, and heavy use of pesticides on foods.

More common bacterial toxins that you might have heard about are botulism from *clostridium botulinum*, or staphylococcal infection from *staphylococcus aureus*. Many foods can be involved, but raw milk has been frequently implicated as well as spoiled home-canned foods.

Viral-borne disease is rare, but *hepatitis A*, *Q fever*, and *poliomyelitis* have been a concern in past years. When they do occur, they are associated with infected food handlers (hepatitis A) or stem from contaminated water (poliomyelitis and Q fever).

Parasitic infections can originate from many sources, but fortunately are rare in occurrence. Eating raw or uncooked meat or seafood is usually associated with these outbreaks. Steak tartare lovers, take note.

Med Meaning

Hepatitis is inflammation of the liver, usually caused by a viral infection. **Hepatitis A** is caused by infection with a virus called an *Enterovirus,* and is spread by exposure to contaminated food or water. **Q Fever** is an infection caused by inhaling a small amount of *Rickettsia Coxiella burnatii.* This comes from animals infected by a tick carrying the disease. Rickettsia, a genus of bacteria found in lice, fleas, ticks, or mites, can cause Q Fever and Rocky Mountain Spotted Fever. **Poliomyelitis** is a viral infection that causes damage to the gray matter portion of the brain and brain stem.

Crop Watch

Food contamination with mold or fungi is yet another source of medical problems. The molds can produce toxins called *mycotoxins.* One type of mycotoxin, called *aflatoxin,* may be found on peanuts, tree nuts, almonds, grains, or figs. These toxins can have serious side effects, including loss of appetite, weight loss, and liver damage, or they may even cause fatality.

The fungi can also create a chemical that may be found on grains. In this case, the symptoms include headache, dizziness, chills, nausea, vomiting, and blurred vision. These problems are usually prevented by close observation of crops and destruction of any contaminated grain.

Fishy Poisons

Specifically, the most common foods reported in food-poisoning incidents are seafood or shellfish that contain toxic algae. Oysters can ingest microorganisms such as the hepatitis virus. Thus, they can create concentrated amounts of toxins in their tissue. Eating raw oysters, then, can be a real risk.

Another common source of poisoning comes from scombroid fish, ciguatera, and paralytic shellfish. Scombroid fish poisoning has been discussed earlier, and involves toxic levels of histamine in the fish, caused by not refrigerating immediately after the catch, or not keeping it properly refrigerated afterwards.

Eating fish or shellfish that have high, harmful levels of a toxin produced by algae called *dinoflagellates* causes ciguatera and paralytic shellfish poisoning. Ciguatera can be found in fresh reef fish such as grouper, snapper, and barracuda. This occurs only if the fish have ingested large amounts of algal toxin. This problem is endemic in Hawaii and Florida. The toxin is not destroyed by cooking, and is found in largest amounts in the fish's internal organs. The toxin in shellfish is mostly saxitoxin, and is found in mussels, cockles, clams, and scallops. The problem can be avoided by not harvesting shellfish in posted areas or in areas exposed to a red tide.

Tales of Milk and Honey

An infrequent occurrence results in a situation called *toxic honey*. The toxin involved is called *andromedo toxin*. When bees collect nectar from rhododendrons, azaleas, laurel, jasmine, or nightshade, this toxicity can occur, as these plants contain a dangerous *alkaloid* in the nectar. Fortunately, this condition is very rare, and can be avoided if beekeepers are scrupulous about the source of their honey.

Med Meaning

Alkaloid is a plant product containing nitrogen and possessing pharmacologic activity. Alkaloid names end in -ine such as morphine, atropine, and cholchicine.

Milk sickness is another unusual cause of illness related to drinking cow's milk. This situation occurs when the cows graze on toxic weeds. While this occasionally happens, it is preventable by knowledgeable herdsmen or dairy farmers watching the grazing area.

Last Man on the Food Chain

Man-made pollutants and contaminants do occur and can be man-removable. Industrial waste in the soil—such as aluminum, arsenic, cadmium, cobalt, iron, lead, mercury, and selenium—can enter the food chain in their original form, or be changed by bacteria. These go into the water supply through run-off caused by floods or heavy rain. They can then be found in plankton, which are eaten by fish, which in turn are eaten by humans.

Skulls and Bones

Be mindful of storing acidic foods such as cooked tomatoes in copper, galvanized, or tin containers. This can lead to food poisoning.

Pesticide poisoning is uncommon with the modern washing techniques of products. Nevertheless, when it does occur, all forms of it can make you very sick, and are sometimes mistaken for a food allergy.

My Body Made Me Do It!

Foods don't have to contain toxins in order to make us feel uncomfortable. Our body's own metabolic pathways or internal engine and all of its parts can make a difference in how the body reacts to normal, routine food.

Fad Diets Could Do You In

For example, in some parts of the country, the water and soil are low in iodine. Eating cabbage, which contains chemicals called *goitrogens*, can cause the thyroid to enlarge. For this reason, it's best to purchase table salt with iodine called *iodized table salt*. Excessive salt, however, can cause high blood pressure. Avidin, a vitamin antagonist in raw egg white, can cause a skin problem from biotin deficiency. Synthetic diets with excessive amounts of amino acids can cause nausea or headache. Be very careful of supplements in fad diets.

Deficiency Issues

Another group of people have some type of deficiency in their way of processing nutrients and other parts of the food. Here the food is routine, but creates a problem only because the person is lacking some vital parts of the metabolic process.

Wilson's disease occurs when normal amounts of copper in food become a problem, because the person lacks *ceruloplasmin*. He or she cannot get rid of the copper, so it accumulates in the body tissue.

Celiac disease is one in which individuals are sensitive to gluten.

A diabetic, whose pancreas cannot produce insulin, needs to monitor calorie and sugar intake.

The most important cause of malabsorption of carbohydrate from the intestinal tract is a deficiency of *oligosaccharidase*. This is an inborn error of metabolism appearing early in life, with symptoms of bloating, cramps, rectal gas, and diarrhea. Commonly, these symptoms are mistaken as a food allergy.

Med Meaning

Ceruloplasmin is a transport system in the bloodstream to get rid of copper in foods, as well as other unwanted things that might be introduced into the system.

I Really Miss Ice Cream!

Lactose intolerance seems to be a more frequently recognized problem. As we have seen, in this situation, the person cannot break down the sugar in cow's milk (lactose). It cannot be absorbed, often causing symptoms of bloating, abdominal pain, diarrhea, or constipation.

Most people have low levels of *lactase*, the enzyme necessary to break down lactose, between the ages of 3 years and puberty, especially between 3 and 14 years of age. Drinking even moderate amounts of cow's milk may result in susceptible people having symptoms.

Secondary lactose deficiency can occur in an otherwise healthy person, after having an acute infectious diarrhea. This condition is also associated with people who have chronic bowel problems. The lining of the gut is denuded so that it cannot produce the enzyme lactase. It also cannot make other enzymes such as sucrase or maltase. These persons may also have problems with sugars like sucrose and maltose.

Lactose deficiency may coexist in persons with food allergies that have an effect on the gut wall.

How Green Is My Salad?

In the past 10 or more years, patients with asthma have been faced with a new enemy. The preservative sodium metabisulfite and related compounds can cause severe, if not fatal, reactions in those sensitive to this chemical.

This preservative is inexpensive and commonly used in salads, avocado dip, vinegar, sausages, dried vegetables, dried fruit, soft drinks, fruit juice, cider, beer, wine, and seafood. It is used as a "stay fresh" spray on foods that are on display in restaurants and fruit markets. In one case, it was fed to lobsters in a tank in a restaurant so they would have a bright red appearance.

The exact physiologic manner in which this preservative works to cause problems is not well understood. Exposure can come as inhalation through sulfur dioxide in the air, or simply by opening a container of food that contains this as a preservative. Ingesting the food or beverage causes the same symptoms, which can range anywhere from acute breathing problems to gastrointestinal distress, to hives, or even death in susceptible persons. This situation occurs most commonly in asthmatics.

Sugar Makes Me Crazy!

A prolonged, hotly debated subject is whether too much sugar or a sugar allergy cause problems in children and adults. Abnormal glucose tolerance tests are reported in groups accused of antisocial activity.

Cases of high sugar intake related to poor academic work in school have been reported. Aggressive and restless behavior in hyperactive children, as well as increased activity in normal children, is blamed on diets rich in sugar. This was called a *sugar allergy* or *reactive hypoglycemia*.

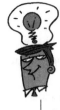

Bet You Didn't Know _____

Remember the "Twinkie defense" murder trial in San Francisco in 1979? The assassin, former San Francisco county supervisor Dan White, claimed he had a sugar high from eating too many Twinkies. He claimed there was a psychological imbalance, which caused him to shoot and kill City Supervisor Harvey Milk and Mayor George Moscone in 1978. White received a voluntary manslaughter conviction and went to jail until 1985, when he was released on parole. He committed suicide almost one year after his release.

However, multiple studies over the past 20 or more years have been unable to prove this theory to be true. Those who made the claims originally relied solely on observations by parents and teachers, not on clinical studies.

True *hypoglycemia* does exist in many forms. It can occur naturally in young children in the first few days of life, especially those of diabetic mothers. Infrequently, it can be caused by tumors of the pancreas.

Reactive hypoglycemia can occur in response to or rebound after sugar-loaded food or *hyperglycemia*. Normally, eating sugar will increase the blood sugar level over one hour. The body then brings it back to normal levels. If no other food is eaten, especially a food high in protein, then the system may over-react, lowering the blood sugar, creating hypoglycemia.

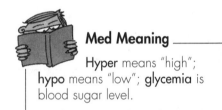

Med Meaning _____

Hyper means "high"; hypo means "low"; glycemia is blood sugar level.

Symptoms of hypoglycemia may include listlessness, confusion, irritability, sweating, increased heart rate, and restlessness. This relatively low blood sugar is very rare and corrects itself to normal in a short period of time. Hypoglycemia is not found after normal meals. Multiple physicians and researchers have looked at children fed different types of sugar and nonsugar substitutes, and found no behavioral or motor changes.

Can't Hold It Together

Food allergies occur when a white blood cell called a *basophil* (in the blood) or *mast cell* (in the tissue) breaks apart (or degranulates) and releases chemicals into the blood-stream. Related chemicals released called *mediators* cause symptoms of the allergy. A true food allergy must involve an immunoglobulin called IgE, which is produced by the person's immune system.

What Goes Around Comes Around

Lectins are chemicals in peanuts, beans, peas, lentils, edible snails, and wheat. These chemicals bind to the mast cell membrane and cause it to break apart, allowing escape of the mediators. (Mast cells are white blood cells that carry chemicals called *mediators* as discussed in Chapter 2.) These chemicals go into the blood stream and cause allergy symptoms.

Ricin is a poison found in kidney beans, which is removed when the beans are soaked and thoroughly cooked. If cooked too slowly or at a low temperature, there will be an increase in the chance for symptoms.

Ricin binds to the lining of the gut wall, allowing nondigested food to leak through into the circulation, where it can start the process of being recognized as foreign material. When these food protein molecules enter the bloodstream, they start a reaction in the immune system with the production of IgE. The next time the food enters the system, the IgE will recognize it and start the process to create an allergic reaction to that food. In other words, it goes around the protected mechanism and enters the bloodstream as too large a molecule. Thus the food allergy process begins.

Med Meaning

Lectin is Latin for choosing. The lectin is very specific for certain carbohydrate molecules on the mast cell surface. If it does not match one, it will not attach.

Binding and Breaking Down

Many foods have other ways of binding to mast cells and causing degranulation. This binding or attachment to the cell membrane is direct, and does not involve IgE. Some foods have peptides, which are protein molecules that bind in this way. These foods include egg whites, strawberries, crustacean shellfish, tomatoes, fish, pork, alcohol, and chocolate. Other foods have an enzyme that breaks down protein, which can also attach to the mast cell membrane and cause a similar reaction.

Foods that contain this enzyme are raw pineapple and papaya, when eaten on an empty stomach. There is no problem with canned pineapple. In the "I don't know" category we have buckwheat, sunflower seeds, mangoes, and mustard, with an as-yet-unrecognized chemical that can trigger the mast cell to degranulate.

It is possible that with ongoing research, these will or have been recently identified.

The Least You Need to Know

◆ Most common symptoms from foods are not caused by an allergy.

◆ Some foods contain histamine or have substances that will produce histamine.

◆ Some foods can cause histamine to be released from mast cells.

◆ Some foods are contaminated with toxins that cause symptoms.

◆ Some people have medical problems that cause them to react to regular foods.

5

SOS: System Failure Alert

In This Chapter

- ◆ Gastroesophageal reflux
- ◆ Laryngopharyngeal reflux
- ◆ Pediatric acid reflux

The body experiences a number of natural reactions when food is introduced into the digestive system. These include the action of the digestion of food in the stomach, with its churning movement, and the activity of acid and other substances called *enzymes* that break down the food. Reactions also involve a nerve called *vagus nerve*, which carries signals to and from the central nervous system. If all goes smoothly, the person has no problems, but on occasion the acid does not stay in the stomach, and the vagus nerve sends the wrong signal. The results of this and the symptoms produced are ofttimes mistakenly thought to be a food allergy. Now the details.

I'm Eating Myself Up

The natural working of the gastrointestinal system, more specifically the stomach, includes the action of acid, which is swishing around to help digest food. Normally, the stomach has a type of lid at the top, called the *gastro-esophageal junction*, which is really a muscle band that contracts to keep the contents of the stomach from escaping back up into the esophagus. Naturally, this muscle relaxes when you eat and swallow, to allow food to slide down the esophagus and empty into the stomach.

The stopper between the stomach and the esophagus doesn't always work effectively, and that means trouble. These problems can involve the lower part of the esophagus, all the way up to the throat. Any and all of our varied apparatus can cause symptoms that mimic allergy problems or are mistaken for food allergies.

The main parts of the digestive system.

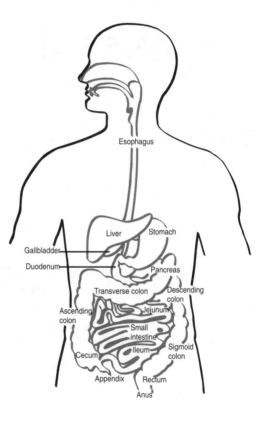

Most people have small amounts of what is commonly known as gastroesophageal acid reflux several times each day. This reflux of acid does not normally cause symptoms. At worst, some people experience mild heartburn symptoms that do not need treatment.

In some people, however, reflux-related symptoms may be so severe that they result in serious physical complications. People who suffer from this condition are said to have *gastroesophageal reflux disease (GERD)*.

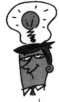

Bet You Didn't Know _____

Your stomach is famous for its acid. Yet acid is only one of four chemicals in the stomach. First is mucous, which helps protect the stomach lining from being burned by acid and other chemicals. Second is hydrochloric acid, which kills swallowed organisms, such as bacteria, and starts up an enzyme called *pepsinogen*. This enzyme breaks down certain parts of the food. When pepsinogen is activated, it changes its form and starts the digestion of proteins. Third, hormones, such as gastrin, help control acid production and the churning action of the stomach. Last but not least, also found in the stomach is a protein called *intrinsic factor*, which is necessary for the intestines to absorb vitamin B_{12}.

Grrrr! It's Gotta Be GERD

According to physicians who specialize in problems of the gastrointestinal tract, GERD is defined as ongoing damage to the lining of the esophagus caused by abnormal amounts of stomach contents refluxing up into the esophagus.

Original reports by gastroenterologists going back 15 or more years stated that about 20 percent of the population had symptoms of GERD. Most recently, in the past 3 to 4 years, the feeling by these specialists is that the frequency has doubled. They state that the reason is related to the common finding that the patient with GERD is usually obese, and the incidence of obesity has doubled over that period of time.

Heartburn is the most common symptom associated with GERD, but there are many nonesophageal symptoms. In those patients with cardiac-type chest pain, 30 percent or more have normal coronary arteries. Sixty percent of these patients were found to have acid reflux as the cause, and twenty percent had chronic cough.

Skulls and Bones _____

The classic definition of heartburn is a burning sensation that starts behind the breastbone and moves from under the breastbone toward the neck. Be careful, because this can also be a symptom of a heart attack. Make sure you consult your doctor. The medical term for heartburn is *pyrosis*, which is Greek for "burning."

Additional symptoms include vocal cord nodules, laryngitis, hoarseness, spasms of the throat around the larynx, and voice changes.

The natural history and pathology of this problem is based on acid reflux. Acid reflux is a mechanical problem of the gastroesophageal sphincter, allowing abnormal acid refluxing up into the lower esophagus. There are three possible reasons that this can occur:

- The first possibility is that there is a transient relaxation of the sphincter, which can occur naturally from medication such as theophylin used by asthmatics, or related herbs, or simply in the swallowing process.

- The second reason could be that the sphincter has lost its natural tone or is unable to maintain its tone.

- The third reason is that there is some change in the anatomy of the area in which the esophagus empties into the stomach—called the *esophagastric junction*—such as a *hiatal hernia*.

Med Meaning

Hiatal hernia refers to digestive discomfort caused when part of the stomach moves upward through the esophageal hiatus or opening in the diaphragm. *Hernia* (or rupture) means a protrusion of an organ or tissue through an opening in its surrounding walls, especially in the abdominal region. *Hiatal* is derived from *hiatus*, which means an opening or aperture (like the one on your camera).

The diaphragm, which separates the chest from the abdomen, has openings to allow the esophagus, blood vessels, and nerves to go through. In the case of a hiatal hernia, part of the stomach has ruptured upward through an opening in the diaphragm, known as esophageal hiatus. This occurs more often in middle-aged people, due to the muscular part of the diaphragm becoming less toned and losing its ability to separate the two areas. The most common type of hiatal hernia is sliding. In this situation, part of the stomach slides up through the esophageal hiatus into the chest, when the person is lying down or bending over. The person may feel pain, cough, and become short of breath. However, increase in reflux may also be the result of increasing abdominal pressure, as in bending forward or straining, which also decreases sphincter tone and creates the same common cavity.

Intestinal Signals

The nervous system is organized to detect changes in the internal and external environment, evaluate these changes, and then respond. This is important to know, because a significant number of symptoms are mistaken for being allergic in origin, but really are related to normal body responses involving the nervous system, which spans the entire body and coordinates most functions of the body. One nerve in particular, the vagus nerve, starts in the area of the neck and "wanders" down into the chest, with branches to the lungs. It continues down along the esophagus around in the wall of the stomach, following the intestinal tract to the colic flexure. A long road, covering a lot of important territory.

As a result of the many parts of the body that are controlled by this same vagus nerve, a variety of reactions can occur. The stimulus may be in one area but show up in another. Here are some examples: Food filling up the stomach or stretching the stomach stimulates the vagus nerve. The impulse may go up to the nose and mouth, but also goes along the course of the gastrointestinal tract to the left colic flexure. The stimulus along this direction signals the intestine to move. At the left colic flexure it signals the intestine to move the food down the descending colon and out of the rectum.

A second example involves the blood vessels and heart. Branches of the vagus nerve also control whether the blood vessels dilate. A vaso-vagal response is one in which something stimulates the nerve, which will then send a signal to the blood vessels to dilate. This in turn will drop the blood pressure, causing a person to feel faint and perspire. Commonly, this is caused by fear.

Fear can cause the heart to speed up. The vagus nerve has fibers to the heart muscle. Impulses go to the vagus nerve, then to the blood vessels, and then the response occurs. Having a person in this condition lie down and elevate their legs will reverse the situation as the person relaxes.

When the blood vessels dilate, it causes a large amount of blood to go down into the legs and feet, as well as to organs in the abdomen. Elevating the legs causes the blood to return up to the region of the brain, and raises the blood pressure to normal levels. If the person faints with the vaso-vagal response, he or she will fall to the ground, and then in this prone position, the situation will automatically reverse itself.

Finally, a third example goes up toward the central nervous system, where signals in one nerve "wire" to involve nerves in close proximity. An example of this is the person who has sneezed and has a runny nose just before or during a bowel movement. Again the person may think this is due to a particular food or food allergy. It is not.

Here again, the normal stimulus of the colon will send a signal up to the vagus nerve. The impulse reaching the medulla and pons can stimulate the facial and trigeminal nerve, which causes this natural response. It is not the food; it is the natural process of the body.

There is a group of people who have normal results when undergoing *endoscopic* studies. Endoscopic means using a device such as a telescope that enables the physician to look into a cavity of the body. In this case, we can look down into the esophagus to see if any damage has been done, and if so, exactly where it's occurring.

Fifty percent of patients with GERD show no evidence of damage. These are referred to

Med Meaning

Endoscopy is a medical procedure that uses a device such as a telescope in order to look into a cavity of the body. If you have an acid reflux problem, your doctor can look down into your esophagus to see what's going on, and exactly where in your esophagus the problem is happening.

as having nonerosive reflux disease. Still others have normal acid exposure, but have symptoms. This group is called *hypersensitive* or *acid sensitive esophagus*.

Sneaky Culprits

There is no one absolutely accurate test for diagnosing uncomplicated GERD. Symptoms of heartburn and acid reflux occurring together more commonly point to having GERD. Many symptoms of acid reflux may occur in other parts of the body. You have to be aware of them because they are often mistaken for allergies. Examples include inflammation of the throat, ears or sinuses, accompanied by pain and congestion.

Other symptoms could be vocal cord problems, laryngitis and voice changes, including hoarseness and commonly chronic cough. In the chest, symptoms of asthma, chronic bronchitis, or even pneumonia can occur. Other patients have had generalized chest pain, sleep apnea, and dental erosion.

Villainous Vagus Redux

The vagus nerve comes out of the Central Nervous System (CNS) at a location called *Jugular Foramen* in the neck and sends out branches to muscles of the pharynx; it then leads down into the trachea or breathing tube and into the esophagus, which is the tube that carries food into the stomach.

The main body of the vagus nerve continues snaking its way down the esophagus in the chest. Here, it sends out fibers to areas of the lungs and heart. At the bottom of the esophagus, the vagus nerve continues along through the diaphragm opening and along the stomach to the intestines, and goes all the way to the left bend of the colon.

Other branches of the vagus nerve go to pulmonary blood vessels that allow the vessels to dilate, and to still other branches that cause glands in the lining of the lungs to produce mucus. Other branches go to the area that controls the cough reflex, while still others control the ability of the lungs to expand. Following this nerve through the opening in the diaphragm, we see that it reaches the intestines, and then goes down into the rectum.

Symptoms involving the lungs, such as asthma and chronic cough, involve the wandering vagus nerve. Right and left branches of the vagus nerve travel down the sides of the esophagus. Acid irritation of the esophagus walls also irritates the vagus nerve, sending impulses back upward and through branches of the nerve to the lungs. This in turn can cause spasm in the lungs, which produces symptoms of asthma, including constant coughing and mucus production. This also stimulates the making of increased amounts of saliva and secretions in the throat.

Some people mistake this condition for postnasal drip, thinking the secretions in the throat are dripping down from the sinuses. The person complains of mucus in the throat that needs to be cleared out. When the patient is given decongestants, drying agents, or even antihistamines, these medications don't help. This occurs mainly because the source of the mucus isn't draining down from the sinuses, but is coming up from the lungs or produced right there in the throat.

The problem is neither food nor allergy, but acid reflux.

Eating and Sniffling

Many people will have a runny nose every time they eat, and presume they are having an allergic reaction to the food they're eating. Actually, this is usually not a food allergy, but irritation of a nerve that causes increased secretion of mucus in the nose.

Gustatory rhinitis, or runny nose when eating, occurs in some people every time they eat. The exact cause is unknown, but there are two explanations. One possibility is that the mechanical movement of the jaw in chewing stimulates certain nerves. This in turn stimulates the production of saliva and tears, which drain into the nose through the lacrimal duct.

Another explanation is that food going into the stomach stretches the stomach and stimulates the branches of the vagus nerve, which run along the outside lining of the stomach. This creates an impulse that runs back to the parts of the brain known as the pons and the medulla, where the electrical stimulus will spill over into the root of certain nerves, thereby causing increased mucus in the nose.

A medical student who would always wipe his nose at mealtime claimed this was the only way he would know when his stomach was full. When his nose started to run, he would stop eating.

Amazing signals!

Bad Aspirations, Vicious Cycle

To make matters worse, sometimes coughing can cause the acid to reflux up the esophagus and spill over into the lungs. This is called *aspiration*. This action creates a cycle in which vagus nerve irritation causes the cough; the cough in turn forces acid up out of the stomach to further irritate the vagus nerve, which causes further coughing. This goes on and on in a cough-reflux cycle. In turn, it may set up a situation in which coughing from any cause could create further acid reflux.

Timely Tip

One third to one half of asthma patients with reflux have no other symptoms of GERD. Some clues to this include the starting of asthma in adulthood, no family history of asthma, and wheezing made worse with meals.

Symptoms higher up in the sinuses, ears, and larynx are related to direct acid exposure. This action usually occurs at night, when the protective measures are lowered. Currently, otolaryngologists, specialists in the area of ear, nose, and throat problems, theorize that the stomach acid may actually go up into the area of middle ear, sinuses, and certainly the throat at night, while the person is lying down or sleeping.

Red Alert

Some symptoms are red flashing alarm signals. These include difficulty swallowing, pain on swallowing, weight loss, vomiting blood, or passing blood from the rectum. Such signals mean that a physician should be consulted immediately.

At the other extreme are symptoms that are easily controlled with over-the-counter medications. Some of these symptoms also include increased saliva, bloating, belching, or a feeling of indigestion.

Sometimes something we're taking for other medical conditions (or using for our own pleasure) can make acid reflux worse. Examples include nicotine (you know where that comes from); nitroglycerin for heart patients; theophyllin, used for patients with asthma or other pulmonary problems; blood pressure medicine like calcium channel blockers; antianxiety medication; and drying agents for increased secretions or congestion, to name just a few.

Shall We Test?

Many diagnostic tests are available, but the one recommended is the results of therapeutic approach. A trial of specific medication and lifestyle changes is the most useful diagnostic test. In this case, treatment for acid reflux leading to control or even disappearance of symptoms, is interpreted as a positive diagnosis, meaning that this was the problem.

Other tests such as barium dye x-ray studies have very limited value in uncomplicated GERD. It is most useful in patients complaining of difficulty in swallowing or pain when swallowing. In this case, experts are looking for stricture or malignancy.

The indication for endoscopy or looking directly into the esophagus would be if a patient had the alarm signals already mentioned, in order to look for a potential pre-cancerous condition called *Barrett's esophagus*.

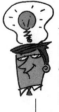

Bet You Didn't Know

The incidence of GERD is increasing in the United States. Medical specialists feel it is because of increased obesity in our population.

Help Me, Please!

Treatment for this condition is divided into two approaches: one is using medication, and the other is changing lifestyle. Occasional symptoms can usually be treated with over-the-counter medication, such as antacids or H2 receptor antagonists.

Hydrochloric acid is produced in the stomach in glands called *gastric glands*. The actual cells that produce this acid are called *parietal cells*. This is one of the things that stimulate the enzyme called *hydrogen/potassium adenosine triphosphate*, more commonly known as the proton pump.

Have Some Meds

Antacids are chemicals such as magnesium hydroxide, aluminum hydroxide, or calcium salts. Troublesome acid is reduced by a chemical action between the antacids and the acid. For example, magnesium hydroxide plus hydrochloric acid (a stomach acid), form magnesium chloride and water. This removes the unwanted acid, and works best if taken between meals.

Other medications, sold over-the-counter, are called *H2 receptor antagonists*. Remember, histamine is one trigger to start the process of acid production. To do this, the histamine has to hook up to a receptor site on the cell that produces the acid. One way to stop acid production would be to block the receptor hookup site of the histamine.

> **Timely Tip**
>
> You can change the amount of acid produced in the stomach by taking medication called *proton pump inhibitors* (PPI). This is the most important medication in treating acid reflux damage to the esophagus. PPIs may need to be taken one or two times daily, and can only be prescribed by physicians.

Examples of medications that accomplish this are Zantac, Pepcid, Tagamet, and Axid. They work best if taken before any activity that would cause acid reflux, such as eating certain foods the patient knows cause problems. H2 receptor antagonists are long acting, while antacids are short-lived. Using the two together could provide short-term, immediate relief, combined with sustained relief.

Proton pump inhibitors such as Prilosec, Previcid, Protonix, and Nexium markedly decrease acid production, since they block acid secretion. They are more effective than H2 receptor antagonists and potentially can work for a full 24 hours.

Skulls and Bones

There is an increased chance of developing esophageal cancer in patients who have untreated esophageal acid reflux. It is extremely important that this be treated and closely watched by a health-care provider.

However, this is not always the case. PPIs do not work on demand, and may take several days to be effective. PPIs are most effective when taken thirty minutes before a meal; in addition, the food to be eaten must contain proteins and/or amino acids. Not taking the medication properly may make it appear that there is no response. It's as if you're knocking on a door, but nobody lets you in.

PPIs have had an excellent safety profile over the past 15 years.

The Times They Are A-Changin'

In treating this problem, it is most important to change your way of living. Taking a pill is easy compared to changing your lifestyle. No medication will be totally effective if the patient will not and does not change certain things in his life, such as detrimental habits.

Timely Tip

Some patients whose conditions are well controlled by medical therapy may be candidates for surgery as an alternative to lifelong medication. This group includes patients with nighttime reflux as well as those with extra esophageal causes, such as hiatal hernia. The best predictor of good response to surgery is good response to medical therapy.

Reflux is usually associated with obesity. Okay, so lose weight. That's easy, isn't it? And it makes a difference (in more ways than one)! Next, avoid reflux-producing food and drink, such as fatty foods, caffeinated drinks, chocolate, coffee, mint, spicy foods, garlic, onions, and tomato-based foods.

Stop smoking and decrease or stop alcohol consumption. Avoid lying down for two to three hours after meals. Sleep with the head of the bed or your upper body elevated about six inches. An easy way is to get a foam rubber wedge to elevate your chest and head. Avoid medications that increase GERD.

Oh, and here's another easy one: Avoid stress!

Stop Clearing Your Throat

As early as 200 C.E., the Roman physician Galen described the gastroesophageal junction and called it *Cardia*. He used this term because symptoms arising from pathology at the gastroesophageal junction mimicked those from heart problems. In 1618, another famous physician, Fabricus, described this junction, and gave it its present name. Finally, in the twentieth century, researchers discovered the relationship of these problems to acid reflux.

In 1890, Chevalier Jackson perfected the light esophascope, so scientists could actually look directly into the parts of the throat and down into the esophagus. Throat symptoms and problems with the larynx, voice box, and the pharynx—the back of the throat—were thought to be related not to acid reflux but to vagus nerve reflex.

Now we know that there are many reasons for these symptoms. These include gastro-esophageal acid reflux, vagus nerve reflex, and a new concept called *laryngopharyngeal reflux (LPR)*. The latter condition can coexist with the other two, or it can exist solely on its own. Until we learned exactly how this came about, throat and voice symptoms were described by many names: extra esophageal reflux, gastro-pharyngeal reflux, laryngeal reflux, supra-esophageal reflux, and reflux laryngitis.

Med Meaning

The word *reflux* comes from the Latin *re*, meaning "back," and *fluxus*, meaning "flow." So **LPR** is back flow of stomach contents into the throat, the larynx, the pharynx, and the esophagus.

It was clear that everyone believed there had to be a relation between GERD and the new condition. After all, how could acid get to the throat without going through the esophagus? It turns out that this is true, but that the acid does not necessarily burn the esophagus on its way up to the throat.

The mystery has been unraveled, and its answer explains why patients can have throat symptoms without esophageal burning.

The Difference Between Night and Day

Comparing the two conditions—LPR versus GERD—shows that LPR is primarily a daytime reflux when the person is upright, while GERD is mainly nighttime, when the person is lying down. Remember, you can have both, but not always. Less than one third of people with LPR also have GERD.

Some researchers feel that increased mucus in the nose and throat is from LPR or vagal response, or even a combination of both. There is even a theory that some middle ear problems are related to LPR. The question asked is: Is there pepsin in the middle ear from gastric acid reflux?

Wouldn't that be interesting? Maybe you've been treating ear symptoms and redness in the ear with antibiotics, when you should have been using medicine to decrease gastric acid.

Lotta LPR

The symptoms of LPR are different from those of GERD. Patients with LPR deny feeling heartburn or feeling stomach contents coming back up into the chest. LPR patients usually complain of hoarseness and throat symptoms such as chronic cough, something being stuck in their throat, chronic throat clearing, changes in their voice, and difficulty in swallowing.

Some people have tabulated symptoms in the order of their frequency. At the top of the list is chronic or intermittent voice changes. Going down the list are vocal fatigue, voice breaks, chronic throat clearing, excessive throat mucus, post nasal drainage, a feeling of something stuck in the throat, heartburn, airway obstruction, spasm of the larynx, and at the bottom of the list is wheezing.

Acid Damages

The diagnosis of LPR is based on symptoms, changes in the area of the throat on examination, and if possible, measuring the *pH* value to see how acidic the secretions are. In GERD, the defect is in the lower esophageal sphincter. In LPR, the defect is in the upper esophageal sphincter. This sphincter lies just below where food enters the esophagus from the throat. It usually stops food from coming back up into the throat after it is swallowed.

Med Meaning

pH is a symbol for the negative logarithm of the hydrogen ion concentration measured in moles per liter. A pH value of more than neutral is called *alkaline* or base, which is the opposite of acidic. A pH value of less than neutral is acid. Neutral is usually a pH of 7.

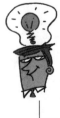

Bet You Didn't Know

Dental enamel exposed to acid from acid reflux will cause dental erosion. The enamel dissolves when exposed to a pH value of less than 3.7.

Important information has been discovered recently. The larynx is one hundred times more sensitive to acid and pepsin injury than the esophagus. The reason for this is that the esophagus has more protective mechanisms. It produces a base material to neutralize the acid, the lining of the esophagus protects it, and movement of the muscle of the esophagus, peristalsis, pushes the stomach reflux so it doesn't stay in one place for a long time.

The most significant factor is that the acid must be of a lower pH, or more acidic, to cause damage in the esophagus, while being less acidic can still damage the larynx and pharynx. Specifically, a less acidic acid reflux could pass through the esophagus without causing damage, but would injure the throat, whereas a more acidic acid reflux can damage the esophagus, the larynx, and the pharynx.

It is estimated that 20 percent of the population have small amounts of reflux every day. Usually this causes hoarseness, voice changes, and laryngitis for a few days. However, a medical specialist should evaluate chronic throat clearing, chronic cough, and difficulty swallowing.

What's the Treatment?

The treatment of LPR is similar to the treatment of GERD, but will require a longer period of time, usually in excess of four to six months. Patients must change their diet, lose weight, and stop smoking. All of these recommendations are the same suggestions as with the treatment of GERD. The medications used are the same, including the H2 receptor antagonists such as Zantac or Tagamet, and proton pump inhibitors, such as Prilosec or Protonex.

Usually in cases LPR, the patient needs these medications in larger amounts more frequently, as well as for longer periods of time.

Even the Children

As early as 1892, physician Sir William Osler was observing that there was some relation between acid reflux and asthma. Other researchers after him thought that LPR was more common in children than adults, because in infants and children the protection of the lower esophageal sphincter was not fully developed. In addition to this, the length of the esophagus is obviously shorter in children than in adults.

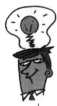

Bet You Didn't Know

Sir William Osler (1849–1919) was the best-known physician in the English-speaking world at the turn of the twentieth century. Canadian-born, McGill-trained, Dr. Osler was the first Professor of Medicine at Johns Hopkins. He has been called the "most influential physician in history" as well as the "father of psychosomatic medicine." The training program he developed for physicians is still followed in medical schools today. He later moved to England, where he held the Regius Chair in medicine until his death.

Gerber Babies' GERD

Esophageal reflux is found in children, and is divided into different categories. The first category is called *physiologic*, and includes infrequent vomiting with no other abnormalities found. The condition does not cause symptoms, rarely occurs during sleep, and often happens while an infant is upright after having eaten. Every parent burps their baby with a towel or diaper on the shoulder. Usually the baby will spit up after eating, so all parents are familiar with this activity.

Another group of infants is said to have pathologic GERD, a condition which causes problems in the intestinal and respiratory tracts. (These symptoms will be covered later in this chapter.)

Long-Term LPR?

Esophageal reflux is self-limited—it will clear up with time. The problem usually gets better by the end of the first year of life, when there is a change from a liquid to a solid diet. Most newborns and infants have reflux after eating. However, if there is long-term reflux—when a child is older than three years of age—then there can be complications.

Clinical complications in the first year of life include failure to grow and failure to thrive. Additional problems can occur in the airways. These may include recurrent bronchitis, croup, pneumonia, and chronic asthma.

The effect of reflux of food and/or stomach acid could happen in one of many ways. One would be aspiration of gastric content into the lungs, causing a type of chemical lung inflammation. Another would be the stimulation of the vagal nerve complex that causes constriction of the bronchial tubes.

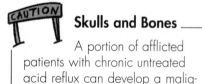

Skulls and Bones

A portion of afflicted patients with chronic untreated acid reflux can develop a malignancy of the esophagus.

Surgery is reserved for those cases in which aggressive nonsurgical therapy hasn't worked and there are serious complications of the reflux noted.

Life-Threatening LPR

A small group of children with asthma or chronic cough that fails to improve with standard medical treatment should be suspected of having LPR. The chronic cough itself will increase pressure within the abdomen, which in turn will cause acid reflux. This then could lead to chronic laryngitis and a wet-sounding voice or cough.

The most serious effects can be apparent life-threatening events. Cases have been reported of periods in which infants stopped breathing (apnea), and had slowing of the heartbeat (bradycardia). Actually, one of the theories for the cause of sudden infant death syndrome (SIDS) is acid reflux that affects the heartbeat and breathing.

Up and Out of the Stomach

The other end of the stomach is called the *pylorus*. After food is churned, exposing it to enzymes and other digestants, it is pushed by the muscles, contracting and relaxing into and through the pylorus, the part of the body where the food leaves the stomach, into the intestines. This movement is called *peristalsis,* as it moves the food along into and through the intestinal tract.

A condition known as pylorospasm in infants occurs most commonly between two and twelve weeks of age. This happens when the area of smooth muscle fiber fails to relax, and a muscle spasm occurs at the exit door of the stomach. Food does not pass through, backs up, and watch out—vomiting occurs. Eventually the muscle relaxes, either naturally or with medicine, and all is well. Sometimes this vomiting, which is natural in this situation, is mistaken for a food allergy.

Congenital hypertrophic pyloric stenosis is another pyloric condition not to wish for. This particular problem is different, in that it is not a muscle spasm. Instead, here the muscle of the pylorus is thickened right at the time of birth. This happens to 1 out of 150 male infants and to 1 out of 750 female infants.

In this situation, the canal or opening is narrowed so that little or no food can get through. Again, vomiting occurs, but the emesis comes out in such force that it is called *projectile vomiting*. In such instances, the food may virtually be shot across the room. Projectile vomiting is one symptom to make us suspicious that we're not dealing with a food allergy; instead, the problem may be a congenital anomaly running in families.

Diagnosing Infant Acid Reflux

How does anyone make a diagnosis of LPR in an infant or child? Both doctor and parents should pay attention to the infant's history at birth and immediately following birth, especially if there are feeding and airway problems. Acid reflux should be suspected if the following occurs:

- Frequent vomiting that is always related to meals
- Associated breathing problems
- Nervous system problems
- Poor weight gain

One way to see if there is damage to the esophagus is to look directly through an instrument called a *fiber optic laryngoscope*. This instrument can detect abnormalities such as foreign bodies, infection, and other conditions. Endoscopy, or looking directly into an area with a scope, allows the doctor to see directly any changes in the esophageal lining.

Choices and Changes

If the physician is suspicious or can prove that the patient has the problem, then there are three choices for treatment. They are lifestyle changes, treatment with medication, or if really necessary, surgery. The amount of treatment is determined by the amount of acid reflux. Many infants and older children respond well to lifestyle changes.

Conservative treatment includes raising the head of the bed; thickening the milk; avoiding foods that would lower the tone of the esophageal sphincter; and not feeding at or just before bedtime. Propping a bottle with the infant lying flat is probably not a good idea.

If none of this works, medication should be considered. Medication is usually helpful, although many of the standard adult medications for this condition are not approved by the FDA for use in infants.

The Least You Need to Know

♦ Acid reflux is becoming a more common problem in today's world.

♦ Specialists in the field feel increased instances of acid reflux are related to increased incidence of obesity in the population.

♦ A portion of afflicted patients can develop a malignancy of the esophagus.

♦ GERD and LPR can exist without symptoms of heartburn.

♦ Some throat and breathing problems can be caused by or made worse by acid reflux.

♦ Successful treatment usually includes a lifestyle change and a diet, along with medication.

Chapter 6

Meet the Usual Suspects

In This Chapter

◆ Learn what a real food allergy is

◆ Discover food allergy's relation to immunoglobulins

◆ Take stock of the most common food allergies

◆ See what's on the list in food groups

After understanding what causes a true food allergy, you need to know which foods to be most wary of. The most common foods that are observed to be problems are eggs, cow's milk, peanuts, and fish in childhood years. Later, as we approach teenage and adult years, other foods are added to the list, including shellfish, tree nuts, and grains such as wheat and corn. Naturally, this is not an inclusive list, but one of foods that are most common. (For a more detailed listing, read on.) The added information needed includes other foods in the same food family that react and also cause allergy symptoms.

A True Food Allergy

According to a report of the National Institute of Allergy and Infectious Disease and the American Academy of Allergy, Asthma, and Immunology, the definition of a food allergy is as follows:

A food allergy or hypersensitivity is an immunologic reaction resulting from the eating of a particular food or food additive. This occurs only in some patients and can happen after eating only a small amount of the food. The reaction is not related to chemical or physiologic effect of the food on the body.

A food allergy is the immune system reacting to a food that it has been programmed to interpret as being a foreign, harmful invader. It does this through producing antibodies that are specific for that specific food the next time the person eats the food. The specific immunoglobulin recognizes it and starts a reaction involving many blood cells. Eventually in the chain of events, large amounts of chemicals called *mediators* are released into the tissues. These chemicals, which include histamine, create multiple allergic symptoms, depending on the location of the allergic reaction.

Most frequently the immunoglobulin involved is IgE. This reaction occurs in a very short period of time after eating the offending food, and is called an *immediate reaction*. Other reactions can involve IgG, IgM, IgA, and S-IgA. These can occur at a later time and are called *delayed reactions*. The immunoglobulin antibodies react with the allergen and the mast cell or basophil, which release their deadly chemicals, until finally the result is removal of the food molecule, but with damage to almost everything in the area.

The immunoglobulin molecule is a protein in the shape of a Y. The stem region is important because its structure can vary, its particular structure or arrangement deciding whether it will be IgG, IgE, IgA, IgM, or IgD. The arms of the Y structure are called *variable*, because component parts vary so that each antibody can hook on to a different, specific antigen. That's what makes it a specific antibody for a specific molecule.

Imagine these antibodies swimming freely in the bloodstream, all looking for a specific food molecule. Or imagine the stem part of the Y hooked onto the surface of a mast cell or basophil cell, its arms waving, trying to attract the food molecule it's seeking. All immunoglobulin basic shapes are the same. Two IgA molecules hook together with a J piece to form S-IgA in the secretions. IgM has multiple J pieces and actually five of them join together. A J piece is a molecule that connects two IgA immunoglobulins together, and in the case of IgM, there are four J pieces that join together five IgM immunoglobulin molecules.

Of Major and Minor Food Allergens

Food allergens are not loners; they come in groups. And whatever their differences may be, they do have one thing in common—a type of protein called a *glycoprotein*. It is large in size, by molecular standards, weighing between 10,000 and 60,000 daltons, which is many million times lighter than an ounce. (A dalton is an atomic mass unit.)

So-called major food allergens are heat stable—which means they are not changed with heat processing—resistant to acid, and resistant to the breakdown by the enzyme *proteasis*.

Major food allergens such as milk, fish, some protein parts of eggs, or peanuts in very small amounts in a natural, cooked, or processed form, can cause symptoms in a sensitized person. Minor food allergens include fresh fruits and vegetables that cross-react with pollen in the oral allergy syndrome. These allergens are heat liable, which means they change with exposure to heat; hence some people who are sensitive to fresh, raw apples can nevertheless eat apple pie without a problem.

Med Meaning _____

Proteases are enzymes that break down protein.

Bet You Didn't Know _____

A study has shown that a short microwave exposure to fresh fruit is enough to change or denature the allergic part, so that it can be eaten without problems by a person who usually develops symptoms from fresh fruit.

Recognize the Prime Offenders

Individual foods that cause allergies are each unique, but share the fact that they have some protein that causes the allergic reaction. It would be wonderful if we could make the food without that part. (Actually some people are trying to create peanuts without the allergic portion.)

Milk

Cow's milk allergy occurs in 2 to 3 percent of children in the first two years of life; 85 to 90 percent of these youngsters will go into remission by 5 to 7 years of age. Cow's milk has at least 20 protein parts. It is usually divided into casein and whey. (Remember Miss Muffet eating her curds and whey?) Casein is between 76 to 86 percent protein. The whey portion has 6 or more proteins, which are not denatured by pasteurization. The most common portion is beta-lactoglobulin.

There are many hidden sources of milk that must be looked for by the person who is allergic to milk. Some brands of canned tuna fish contain a milk protein called *casein;* some processed meats contain casein as a binder, and in some cases, so-called nondairy products also contain casein. (For more information on hidden sources of milk, see Chapter 13.)

Pediatricians might once have commonly suggested goat's milk for a child who was allergic to cow's milk. Now we know that 50 percent of people allergic to cow's milk are also allergic to goat's milk—live and learn. On the other hand, some ingredients in canned food are not milk-related, even though it sounds like they may be. Examples are calcium lactate, calcium stearoyl lactylate, lactic acid, sodium lactate, and sodium stearoyl lactylate. Yet another study reveals that 20 percent of children who were allergic to cow's milk were also allergic to beef.

> **Skulls and Bones**
>
> Choose wisely at the deli counter. The staff may be using the same equipment to cut meats and cheese.

Eggs

Eggs are a common source of protein in our diet: eggs in cooking, eggs for breakfast in many forms, and egg whites, now that we are cholesterol conscious. For the egg-allergic person this is bad news, because egg-sensitive persons usually react only to the egg white portion. The egg white is mostly *ovalbumin*, which is changed by heating or cooking. Yet a part of the egg white, about 4 percent, is *ovomucoid*; it is the most allergenic part and is not heat liable.

Furthermore, researchers have found in the blood of egg-allergic persons IgE antibodies specific to egg yolk and egg white. An egg allergy is common in people allergic to chicken, and these same individuals can have allergies to other birds, such as turkey, squab, guinea hen, partridge, and so on.

> **Med Meaning**
>
> **Ovalbumin** and **ovomucoid** are protein portions of the egg and are found in egg white.

> **Skulls and Bones**
>
> It is very important to read food labels. Some noodle pastas might read "yolk free," but remember, the egg white can be the demon.

Eggs are an ingredient in many foods and drinks. On some bar drinks or coffee drinks, there is a foam or milk topping—this might contain egg. Most egg substitutes contain some egg white. Some pastas, including those in soups, contain egg. And of course, don't forget stracciatella and egg drop soups.

The American Academy of Pediatrics and Allergy Associations agree that the measles, mumps, and rubella (MMR) vaccine can be safely given to patients with egg allergy. A recent article shows that the same thing is true of the flu vaccine.

Peanuts

The major storage proteins of peanuts are *arachin* and *conarachin*. However, the major peanut allergen is called *peanut-I*. Peanuts represent one of the most allergenic foods. Even processed peanut products retain their allergenicity. There is some question as to how safe peanut oil is to allergic people.

Because peanuts are a legume, they can be used in artificial nut preparations. The taste is chemically removed, then the product reflavored with taste of walnuts or pecans. Many foods prepared in ethnic restaurants such as Chinese, Indonesian, Thai, and Vietnamese contain peanuts in some form, or are cross-contaminated during cooking. This can also happen in bakeries and on equipment that produces foods with sunflower seeds and later, peanuts.

Experts suggest that people allergic to peanuts also avoid tree nuts. Some gourmet oils are really cold-pressed, expelled, or extruded peanut oil and should be avoided. You must check the labels on all foods. Many patients ask if children outgrow this allergy. One study says that 20 percent do seem to lose the allergy. More commonly, however, it appears to be a life-long problem.

The good news is that researchers are publishing articles that indicate there is hope on two fronts. One anticipated event is a method to desensitize peanut-allergic patients, while another is developing peanuts without the allergic component. Hopefully, one or both methods will be available, successful, and safe in the future.

Bet You Didn't Know _____

There are many hidden sources of peanuts. Most recently you have probably noticed that conscientious manufacturers are putting warning notices on products that state there could have been some contact with utensils used for peanut products, even though there is no peanut ingredient in the product.

Bet You Didn't Know _____

Mandolonas are peanuts soaked in almond flavor, and arachis oil is peanut oil.

Skulls and Bones _____

Peanuts as well as tree nuts can cause severe life-threatening allergic reactions. It is strongly advised that allergic patients have epinephrine or adrenaline available at all times in case of a generalized anaphylactic reaction.

Peanuts, Tree Nuts—What's Driving You Nuts?

At many social events and bars, one can expect to be served tree nuts and peanuts. For your understanding, it is important to know the difference between a peanut and a tree nut.

Peanuts are a legume, just like peas, lentils, and beans. These grow in the ground. Tree nuts, which include walnuts, Brazil nuts, cashews, filberts/hazelnuts, hickory, pecan, pine, and pistachio nuts, are not peanuts. Tree nuts grow on trees.

Almonds, which are considered a tree nut, are really in the peach family, along with foods such as peaches, plums, cherries, apricots, and nectarines. So those who are allergic to tree nuts must ask, "Is this really a tree nut?"

Because allergic reactions to tree nuts can be so severe, the allergic patient must be aware of hidden sources. Tree nuts have been used in many types of food, such as cereals, crackers, ice cream, and even barbecue sauce. They have been found in natural and artificial flavorings as well.

In the nonfood category, crushed nutshells have been found in beanbags, kicker sacks, and other products of that nature.

How about coconuts that grow on trees? Are they really tree nuts? The coconut is actually the seed of a fruit, so it is not a troublemaker. However, there have been reports of people having allergic reactions, so be careful if you add it to your diet. Some also question nutmeg, which grows on a tropical tree. Nutmeg is considered safe for patients with tree nut allergies.

Soy

Soy is the perfect protein extender. Remember Hamburger Helper? Well, that was the start. Now soy is everywhere in foods and food supplements. All factions of soy are allergenic, one no more than another. Soy is made of globulin and whey factions. The allergy-causing protein parts are heat stable. Avoiding soy is very difficult, because it is in so many foods.

Because pure soy is considered a natural source of estrogen, cancer specialists manage its use in two ways. Women with breast cancer are advised to avoid soy because some breast cancers are made worse with estrogen. We are not talking about occasional consumption of a food with some soy in it, but large amounts of soy, such as a soy supplement.

Men, on the other hand, are encouraged to eat soy, because prostate cancer is decreased or more easily controlled with estrogen or estrogenlike treatment. CapCure, an organization devoted to research and education regarding prostate cancer, publishes recipe books suggesting soy use in many menus.

Soy appears in many products, so you must read the labels. Soy is found in baked goods, canned tuna, crackers, cereals, sauces, soups, and infant formula. A recent report of 20 people given 4 to 8 spoonfuls of soy protein supplement dissolved in water had severe allergic symptoms within 10 to 30 minutes of ingestion. Soy is a very common ingredient in products triggered for weight reduction and body-building.

Shellfish

A reaction to shellfish in the allergic person can be as minor as itching, welts, and swollen lips, all the way to severe abdominal pain, cramping, vomiting, and diarrhea.

Part of the confusion about recognizing a shellfish allergy is that there are two distinct groups of shellfish—crustaceans (which include shrimp, lobster, crab, squid, crayfish, and prawns), and mollusks (which include abalone, mussels, oysters, scallops, clams, snails, squid, and octopus).

Patients may be suspicious because shrimp caused a problem, but clams did not. These patients declare they're not allergic to shellfish, yet they are, but only to one group of shellfish and not the other. There's a 75 percent chance of being allergic to another shellfish within the same group, but a lower percentage of being allergic to the other group. There's a strong chance that if you're allergic to shrimp, you could be allergic to crab and lobster as well, because they are all crustaceans. However, you might not be allergic to members of the mollusk group.

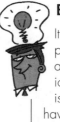

Bet You Didn't Know

It's a common mistake to think people allergic to shellfish are allergic to iodine. Allergy to iodine or radio-contrast material is unrelated to shellfish; the two have no connection to each other. Each food allergy exists, but does not cross-react with the other.

Wheat

Wheat is a grain that really is a cultivated grass. In 20 percent of patients, wheat will cross-react with other grains, such as barley and rye. Some cross-react with oats, rice, or corn. The response to a true wheat allergy is through IgE reacting to the wheat protein glutenin.

Bakers and distillery workers exposed to grain can develop baker's asthma from inhaling wheat, thus having an allergic reaction in the lungs. Other allergic people have gastrointestinal symptoms, increased asthma, or worsened eczema.

Timely Tip

Kamut and spelt are cereal grains and can cause problems. These are commonly used in ethnic and health food restaurants.

Some hot dogs and ice cream contain wheat. Imitation crab and processed meats (sausage, salami, bologna) can also contain wheat. Be aware that many dried flower arrangements and wreaths contain wheat products.

Down Another Pathway—Allergy or Not?

A food allergy can also be defined by some people as reactions to food that involve other immunoglobulins. These are not strict IgE-mediated immediate responses, but some feel any immunoglobulin involvement should be considered an allergy. The reactions to be mentioned next are not immediate, but develop over a longer period of time. Therefore, some refer to these as delayed reaction. This debate goes on.

Food-induced colitis usually occurs at two to three months of age. It is related to cow's milk or soy ingestion. The infant does not appear sick, but has blood in the stool. This usually disappears by six months to two years of age. During this time, the infant should not be fed cow's milk or soy milk, once the diagnosis is made.

Nonceliac malabsorption occurs at ages one to three months. The cause can be related to cow's milk, soy, eggs, or wheat. In these cases, increased IgA and IgG are found.

Celiac disease is more extensive, leading to poor absorption by the gastrointestinal tract. It seems to be hereditary. The cause is a reaction to gliadin, a part of gluten, found in wheat, oats, rye, and barley. The patient has increased amounts of IgA, IgM, and IgG. A small number of patients have increased IgE, and have positive skin test reactions and positive *RAST* blood test. Most patients will outgrow the allergy, but not those with true celiac disease.

Dermatitis herpetaformis is a skin condition in which the patient has an itchy rash, gluten sensitivity, and medical problems with the gastrointestinal tract. The rash is chronic and looks like raised water-filled bubbles. A term for this is *papulovesicular*. It appears evenly on both sides of the body, including the buttocks. Eliminate gluten from the diet, and the rash is gone. In this case, S-IgA is found in the fluid in the rash. The feeling is that the S-IgA comes from the gut.

Other food-related problems might exist. Migraine headaches are sometimes listed as food related, although there is no absolute proof as yet. In one study, 15 percent of 80 patients with migraine headaches saw their headaches disappear on food elimination diets. The same result has been reported with groups of patients with epilepsy.

Seeds

A number of years ago, an allergist reported a series of patients who experienced allergic reactions when eating pizza. Everyone thought this was either a tomato or cheese allergy; however, it turned out the allergic people were able to eat both tomatoes and cheese without a hitch. After exhaustive trial and elimination diets, it came down to one common ingredient. That ingredient was mustard seed, which was used for taste enhancement in the cooking process.

As mentioned in Chapter 1, a small group of foods are responsible for some 90 percent of food allergy reactions. The other 10 percent are caused by about 160 other foods, including seeds such as sesame, sunflower, and poppy. Reactions to seeds can range from mild itching and hives all the way to generalized, life-threatening reactions, including shock and even death.

Seeds are used in preparation of many foods, especially in the baking of muffins, cookies, breads, and cakes. Some are found in crackers and trail mix. Cottonseed in cottonseed oil is discussed separately. To make matters more difficult, extracts of seeds are used in products of the cosmetic line, but will go unrecognized unless mentioned on the label. Examples are shampoos, hair conditioners, lotions, styling products, and facial creams. This can cause problems, whether eaten in the form of food or rubbed onto the skin.

Bet You Didn't Know

Anything that goes on or into your body through any body orifice can cause an allergic reaction.

Let's talk about those oils from seeds. Seed oil, including cottonseed oil, is used in cooking. Most seed oils are highly refined in a process in which most, if not all, of the protein is removed. Included are cottonseed and sunflower oils. Lacking the protein part, there should be no allergic reaction. However, some seed oils are not highly refined, retain the protein, and represent a potential calamity waiting to happen. Again, read the label and hope that the seed is listed, not simply called a spice or additive.

From Bagels to Burgers

A patient did her own detective work. She would break out in hives whenever going to a fast food hamburger stand. At first she surmised the problem must be caused by the dressing or special sauce used on the burger, but noticed the reaction happened only when she ate one particular kind of bun—a sesame seed bun. It appears that fast food restaurants are offering sesame seed buns more commonly these days; hence, more exposure and maybe more allergic reactions.

An interesting observation by those in the baking business, especially bagel stores, is that many times a plain water bagel is dumped into a container that previously held egg bagels or bagels with seeds. This may be done without thoroughly cleaning the bin, but even when the bin is cleaned, a seed or two may be left behind and can adhere to the so-called plain water bagel. Be aware, the same thing happens when breads, cakes, and cookies are moved from tray to tray during the business day.

Remember cross-reactions of foods with latex allergy? As we mentioned earlier, persons who have allergic reactions to latex may also react to bananas, avocados, and kiwis. Birch tree pollen is also considered in this mix. A recent article in an allergy journal has noted a specific protein allergen called *70-kDa protein*. We're closing in fast, and learning more each day.

A protein called *Lipod transfer protein* is found throughout plant foods, in fruits, seeds, and pollen. See how this whole thing fits together? A recent study noted finding these heat-stable substances. Another food with similar allergic protein is onion.

All in the Food Family

If you are allergic to one food, be sure you are aware of all the foods in that group. If you are allergic to one food, you may also be allergic to another food in the same family, because they share similar proteins. Here is a list to help you identify what to look for:

- **Dairy products (cow and goat).** Butter, buttermilk, casein, cheese, cream, ice cream, lactalbumin, milk, yogurt, and some infant formulas.

- **Eggs.** White, whole, and yolk (from chicken, duck, or goose).

- **Fish and shellfish.** This group can be classified into these three families:

  - **Fish.** Anchovy, barracuda, black bass, bluefish, bonito, bullhead, butterfish, carp, catfish, caviar, cod, crappie, croaker, drum, eel, flounder, grayling, grouper, haddock, hake, halibut, harvest fish, herring, mackerel, mullet, muskellunge, perch, pickerel, pike, pollack, pompano, porgy, red snapper, redfish, rockfish, salmon, sardine, scrod, sea trout, shad, smelt, sole, sprat, Sturgeon, sunfish, swordfish, trout, tuna, weakfish, white bass, whitefish.

  - **Crustaceans.** Crab, crayfish, lobster, prawn, and shrimp.

  - **Mollusks.** Abalone, clam, cockle, escargot, mussel, octopus, oyster, quahog, scallop, and squid.

- **Fruit.** This group can be broken down into these families:

  - **Apple.** Apples, cider, apple cider vinegar, crabapple, pear, quince, and quince seed.

  - **Banana.** Banana and plantain.

  - **Citrus.** Citron, grapefruit, kumquat, lemon, lime, orange, tangelo, and tangerine.

  - **Grape.** Champagne, grape, grape wine, raisin, and wine vinegar.

- **Melon.** Cantaloupe, casaba, Chinese watermelon, citron melon, cucumber, gherkin, honeydew melon, muskmelon, Persian melon, pumpkin, summer squash, watermelon, and winter squash.

- **Palm.** Cabbage palm, coconut, and date.

- **Papaya.** Papain and papaya.

- **Heath.** Black huckleberry, blueberry, cranberry, and wintergreen or pyrola.

- **Honeysuckle.** Elderberry.

- **Mulberry.** Breadfruit, breadnut, fig, and hop.

- **Pineapple.** Pineapple. Note: pineapple is listed as a separate family.

- **Plum.** Almond, apricot, cherry, nectarine, peach, plum, and prune.

- **Olive.** Jasmine and olive.

- **Rose.** Black raspberry, blackberry, boysenberry, dewberry, loganberry, red raspberry, and strawberry.

- **Saxifrage.** Currant and gooseberry.

- **Fungi.** Baker's yeast, brewer's yeast, distiller's yeast, Fleischmann's yeast, lactose fermenting yeast, lager beer, mushroom, truffle.

- **Grass.** Cereals, bamboo, barley, bran, corn, hominy, malt, millet, oat, popcorn, rice, rye, sorghum, sugarcane, triticale, wheat, wheat germ, whole wheat, and wild rice.

- **Legume.** Acacia, alfalfa, black-eyed pea, carob bean (St. John's bread), chickpea (garbanzo), common bean, fava bean, green string bean, jack bean, kidney bean, lentil, licorice, lima bean, mesquite, navy bean, pea, peanut, pinto bean, soybean, tamarind, and tragacanth.

- **Madder.** Coffee.

- **Meat.** This group can be divided into these families:

  - **Poultry.** Chicken, Cornish hen, duck, goose, grouse, guinea hen, partridge, pheasant, pigeon, quail, squab, turkey.

  - **Red meats.** Beef, calf, steer, veal, gelatin, goat, ox, lamb, mutton, rabbit, sweetbreads, boar, sausage, scrapple, sow, squirrel, swine, and venison.

  - **Pig.** Pork, ham, and bacon.

  - **Reptiles.** Alligator, crocodile, rattlesnake, terrapin, and turtles.

- **Nuts.** This group consists of these families:

    - **Beech.** Beechnut, chestnut, and chinquapin.

    - **Birch.** Filbert, hazelnut, and wintergreen.

    - **Cashew.** Cashew, mango, and pistachio.

    - **Cola nut.** Chocolate (cocoa) and cola (kola) nut.

    - **Pine.** Juniper and pine nut (pignola).

    - **Walnut.** Black walnut, butternut, English walnut, hickory nut, and pecan.

- **Spices and herbs.** The following families belong to this group:

    - **Ginger.** Cardamom, East Indian arrowroot, ginger, and turmeric.

    - **Laurel.** Avocado, bay leaf, cinnamon, and sassafras.

    - **Mint.** Balm, basil, catnip, hoarhound, Japanese artichoke, lavender, marjoram, mint, oregano, peppermint, rosemary, sage, savory, spearmint, and thyme.

    - **Myrtle.** Allspice, clove, guava, myrtle, and pimento.

    - **Nutmeg.** Mace and nutmeg.

    - **Orchid.** Vanilla.

    - **Pepper.** Black pepper, white pepper.

- **Tea.** Tea.

- **Vegetables.** This group breaks down into these families:

    - **Buckwheat.** Buckwheat, rhubarb, and sorrel.

    - **Goosefoot.** Beets, lamb's quarters, spinach, and Swiss chard.

    - **Lily.** Aloe, asparagus, chives, garlic, leek, onion, sarsaparilla, and shallot.

    - **Mallow.** Cottonseed, marshmallow, okra (gumbo).

    - **Morning glory.** Sweet potato and yam.

    - **Mustard.** Broccoli, Brussels sprouts, cabbage, cauliflower, collards, garden cress, horseradish, kale, kohlrabi, mustard, radish, rutabaga, turnip, and watercress.

    - **Nightshade.** Bell pepper, cayenne pepper, paprika, red pepper, chili, eggplant, ground cherry, melon pear, potato, strawberry tomato, tobacco, tomato, and tree tomato.

♦ **Parsley.** Anise, caraway, carrot, celeriac, celery, coriander, dill, fennel, parsley, and parsnip.

♦ **Poppy.** Poppy seed.

♦ **Sunflower/Composite.** Absinthe (sagebrush or wormwood), artichoke, chamomile, chicory, dandelion, endive, escarole, Jerusalem artichoke, lettuce, oyster plant, safflower, safflower seed, tansy, and tarragon.

The Least You Need to Know

♦ True food allergies involve immunoglobulins, usually IgE.

♦ The protein part of food, the large molecule, is the important, recognized part in a food allergy.

♦ Allergic symptoms depend on in what part of the body histamine and other mediators are located.

♦ Foods are formed into groups, but usually not all foods in the group will cause problems.

♦ You must be aware of all foods you are eating—so read labels and ask questions.

Part 3

A Visit to Your Allergist

You may need the expert services of a true professional, so here's advice on how to start the ball rolling in the right direction, and what you can expect along the way. Yes, take control … trust your problem to someone who's spent a professional lifetime looking at and solving food allergy and food intolerance problems just like yours. Meet your allergist and find out what he or she can do for you.

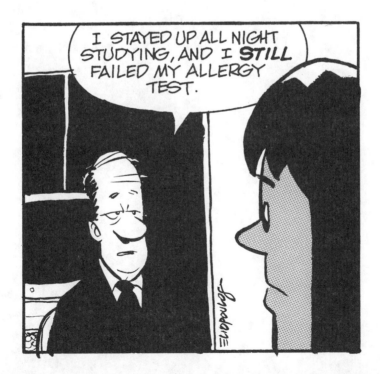

7

The Allergist Is In

In This Chapter

- Find out when you should see an allergist
- Find an allergist that's right for you
- Understand how an allergist focuses on your problem
- Learn what happens during a physical examination

Taking the first tentative step is always the most difficult. People tend to ignore medical symptoms such as a rash or food-induced asthma with a shrug of the shoulders and tell themselves, "It's nothing; it will go away." Most of the time this is true. The sneezing, the stuffy nose, the itchy eyes will disappear with time. If the symptoms continue, an over-the-counter medication may give enough temporary relief, provided there are no apparent or hidden side effects.

However, if you can't find relief, or worse, if your problem starts interfering with your normal activities or sleep, you have to bite the bullet and seek some expert advice from a qualified and trained individual—you have to go and see an allergist. In this chapter, you'll learn under which conditions you should consider seeking expert advice, what to look for in a conventional allergist, and what to expect from a visit to your doctor's office.

When You Should See an Allergist

Making the decision to get advice from an allergist will differ with each person. In general, you should see an allergist if you experience one or more of the following problems:

- When the symptoms of your food allergy and/or inhalant allergy are so severe that they interfere with your daily life, sleep, school, or work.

- When a symptom does not come under control with safe, over-the-counter, or prescribed medications.

- When food allergies or inhalant allergies are creating breathing problems such as asthma or poorly controlled eczema.

- When the medication suggested for these allergy problems causes side effects that interfere with daytime or sleep patterns.

- When you need help in identifying whether this is a food allergy and which foods may be causing the problem.

Timely Tip

Some health-care plans require that you first see your primary care health provider before consulting an allergy specialist. When symptoms are not improving with time or first-line medicines, it is time to request an evaluation by a person trained in diagnosing and treating allergies.

You may also want to see an allergist for these reasons:

- To gather information about a food allergy; to help identify specific foods that might be bothering you; and to gain knowledge about allergy problems that seem to be related to foods, but are really related to food additives or contaminants.

- To get help in identifying foods in their many forms and with many names so they can be eliminated from your diet.

Consider Your Options

Every year, millions of people in North America spend billions of dollars on allergy treatments. Treatment options vary from appropriate to useless and even risky, and can be split into three disciplines—conventional, alternative, and environmental medicine—each advocating its own views on the causes of allergies and how to diagnose and treat them.

◆ **Conventional medicine.** Conventional or traditionally trained allergists maintain that allergies are recognizable immune-system reactions. They rely on three key forms of allergy treatment: avoidance of the substances that are bothering the patient; drugs; and, for selected allergies, immunotherapy (or allergy shots) only in selected and appropriate cases. A conventional or traditionally trained allergist is first trained in a general medicine specialty, such as pediatrics or internal medicine. Next he or she must complete a training program in adult and pediatric allergy. The background in general medicine helps the allergist to recognize medical problems that present themselves with allergylike symptoms.

◆ **Alternative medicine.** Alternative medicine practitioners view allergies as imbalances in the patient's equilibrium. They do not necessarily have the same formal training as conventional allergists. Even if they have received general medical training, their mode of diagnosis and/or treatment is vastly different and not without controversy. The treatment regimen relies on the use of herbal substances and vitamins that are considered to be foods, which are not regulated or standardized by anyone. The treatment program includes very large doses of vitamins and/or herbs which are used to "cleanse your system." This is followed with a program of supplements, additional herbs, and vitamins.

◆ **Environmental medicine.** Environmental medicine doctors argue that whether or not a patient develops allergies depends mostly on factors in the patient's environment. Their treatment regimens are very limiting, if not controversial. For example, patients must wear certain types of clothing, live under confined conditions, eat a prescribed diet, and almost totally separate themselves from their environment.

Both alternative and environmental medicine approaches to testing and treating allergies have been studied repeatedly and have not been clinically proven to be effective or lead to consistent improvement in symptoms for patients. In some cases, alternative approaches have been found to be risky, because they may cause a delay in the diagnosis of serious medical problems. For example, stomach complaints misdiagnosed as a food allergy may turn out to be stomach cancer upon closer examination.

The safest bet in your search for allergy relief is to consult a *board-certified allergist*, who professes the conventional treatment of allergies as sanctioned and recommended by the American College of Allergy and the American Academy of Allergy and Immunology. Depending on the patient, some conventional allergists may endorse alternative therapies as "complementary" allergy treatment in addition to (but not instead of) conventional treatment, if the method may suit or help the patient and does no harm.

Med Meaning

A **board-certified allergist** is a physician who has received three years of formal training in either internal medicine or pediatrics, followed by two or three years of further training in the field of allergy and clinical immunology. In order to earn the designation board-certified allergist, the individual must also pass an examination by the American Board of Allergy and Immunology that tests his or her ability to diagnose and treat allergies in patients. Once certified, specialists must be reexamined every 7 to 10 years to maintain their board certification.

What to Look for in an Allergist

Finding an allergist is not that difficult. Depending on your health-care plan, you may be transferred to a preferred allergist, or you can look up a specialist on the Internet where you can find the names of physicians in your state, as well as information on whether they have been involved in any malpractice lawsuits. Finding an allergist that's right for you, however, also involves the following considerations:

♦ Don't go too far out of your way. Choose an allergist within convenient distance from your home. Usually there are multiple visits, so make your travel time convenient.

♦ Consider carefully the background and accreditation of your allergist; how long has he or she been practicing? Is he or she board certified? You will also want to gauge the doctor's personal qualities.

♦ Trust your instincts. When you meet the allergist, you should be comfortable and feel that he or she is actually hearing what you are saying, giving you answers to your questions, and helping you understand what is happening regarding your allergy symptoms. Making a correct diagnosis takes time and should involve a congenial, yet professional exchange of information.

Timely Tip

If your city has a medical school and an allergy training program, it would be worth a phone call to see which allergists in your city teach in the training program. This usually assures you that this particular allergist is staying current with regard to the latest treatments and therapies.

♦ Check out the support staff. They should show interest in you and give initial information and additional information about your care. They should carefully explain what is planned and what they are doing in the course of your care.

♦ Beware of any warning signs. If what you are being told by the doctor and staff does not make sense to you, then look for another opinion.

Can We Talk?

When you have found the doctor that's right for you, the first thing you'll do is to sit down and have a friendly chat with him or her. Your allergist will question you about the symptoms that cause you discomfort. He or she will also ask you about your family, occupation, hobbies, and personal habits such as smoking and drinking, as well as your home and work environment—all in an effort to get to the root of your problem and give a name to your pain. Remember, your chances of having a true food allergy range anywhere from 2 to 10 percent as the main cause of your problem. This means that more than 90 percent of the time there is another cause for your symptoms, and the answers you provide will help your allergist identify the trigger mechanisms behind your problems. In some cases, the information you provide—commonly referred to as the patient's *medical history*—may be enough for an allergist to make a diagnosis.

What's the Problem?

True food allergies can be very difficult to identify, and patients are not always the best judges of what's bothering them. To get to the bottom of a complaint, an allergist typically will start asking you about the symptoms that are affecting you.

For example, if you are experiencing respiratory (breathing) symptoms of an allergy, your allergist may want to know whether your allergic reaction involves your eyes, ears, and throat only; whether you experience itching, bouts of sneezing, or watery nose and eyes; or whether the symptoms affect only the upper part of your breathing system (your nose and throat, collectively called the *respiratory tree*); or whether the symptoms include your lungs as well.

Food allergies can affect many parts of the body, so they may have many different types of symptoms. As a result, all of these possibilities must be covered by the doctor taking your history.

Next, your allergist will want to get a clear picture of everything surrounding your symptoms. When did they start? How long do they last? Are your symptoms continuous or do they come and go? Did anything change just before the onset of the symptoms—perhaps a new pet, change in diet, new medicine, a move to a new location, any other changes in the household or work place? Do you know of anything that brings on the symptoms, makes them worse, or makes them better? What kinds of things have you tried to help yourself, and do they work?

Timely Tip

You can be proactive in the diagnosis process by keeping a food diary—a detailed record of the foods you eat, including dates, times, and any symptoms observed—that you share with your allergist.

Are You Taking Any Meds?

Many allergy problems start slowly and quietly, so it is important to know about childhood illnesses that might be a sign that allergy problems are on the horizon. Problems or illnesses such as food problems, croup, eczema, seasonal bronchitis, pneumonia, or repeated seasonal hospitalizations are all important.

Likewise, your allergist will want to know whether you are currently being treated for other illnesses, and will ask for a complete list of your medications. In some cases, the medication a patient uses may be involved in the current problem. For example, *beta blockers* used in treating headaches and blood pressure problems may, as a side effect, increase allergic symptoms, especially in asthma. Other medications such as theophylin products used in asthma can increase or even cause GERD or LPR, which in turn can mimic food allergies.

Most people do not pay attention to the medications that are prescribed for them. They rarely remember the names or the strength of the medication. Most physicians' offices provide a wallet-sized card to list all medications currently being used. Also, there should be listed the strength and the dosage schedule. Most important, it should list any medication allergies that the person may have. Again, what the person thinks is a reaction to food, such as a stomachache, diarrhea, bloating, or rash, may actually be due to one of the medications being taken.

Interaction between medications or side effects of the medications are well known, but are not always communicated to the patient by the health-care giver or the pharmacist. Be sure to ask questions if there's anything you don't understand. Usually, both your physician and your pharmacist will check and double-check to see if you have any unanswered questions, and to make sure you know how to use the prescribed medication. You should convey all appropriate information on your medications to your allergist.

Skulls and Bones

Interaction between medications has become such a problem that computers in pharmacies are programmed to alert the pharmacist of a possible adverse interaction between a new medication and others you are taking. For this reason it is important to try to fill all your prescriptions at the same pharmacy or inform the pharmacist of other medications you are taking. At the very least, read the warning label that comes with the medication.

Are Your Reactions Seasonal?

Because a true food allergy occurs only in a small percentage of cases, it is important to get complete information about inhalation allergies that can mimic food allergies. In addition, most people with a food allergy also have an inhalant allergy. Thus it is important to get a complete understanding of what is going on. To that end, your allergist will want to know more details about your chief symptoms: Do they come only during certain parts of the year? Are they apparent all year long? Do they occur all year long, but are worse or better during certain months of the year?

On the East Coast, there are definite seasons with frost or snow on the ground during certain months. This makes an inhalant allergy like pollen allergy more easily recognized as being seasonal. On the West Coast there are pollen seasons, but they meld into each other, so that it is more difficult to get a very specific seasonal history; on the West Coast, something is pollinating all year long. The allergist wants to view the complete patient, not merely one symptom or problem. An example is headaches thought to be from foods may really be due to inhalant allergies, migraines, or medication.

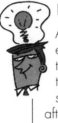

Bet You Didn't Know

Allergens are different in different parts of the country. Moving to a distant location may give the allergy patient one or two symptom-free years. However, after the patient has gone through two pollinating seasons, symptoms may return.

Food allergies are usually not seasonal in nature. They occur when someone is exposed to the food by eating, touching, or inhaling particles. However, reactions may be seasonal if they involve a particular food that is available in great abundance during certain parts of the year, such as certain fruits, types of fish, and shellfish. Kiwi fruit is seasonal, as are avocados. Many times people allergic to latex are also allergic to kiwi and/or avocado. One piece of information may lead to another. What looks like a seasonal problem may be potentially a year-round danger, with certain other exposures, such as latex gloves or the rubber dam used in a dentist's office. Once again, the more information your allergist has, the better the chance to reach an accurate diagnosis about your problem.

Another situation that can arise and appear to be seasonal is a history of melons or strawberries causing problems only when they are in season. This is because the person eats large amounts frequently, which could cause symptoms to occur.

The reason this occurs is because the quantity available is so much greater in season, and the less expensive price allows more people to purchase large quantities. In this

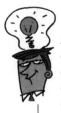

Bet You Didn't Know

Allergic reactions to food are determined by factors such as quantity of the food eaten, frequency of eating the food, and combinations of foods eaten.

case, quantity is the factor that creates the problem. For example, during certain seasons of the year, melons are more plentiful and cheaper. There is more of a chance that a person would buy more and eat more, and this increased amount eaten could trigger allergy symptoms. Other parts of the year, when the food is less plentiful and more expensive, less would be eaten.

Does It Run in Your Family?

The tendency to have allergies is, for the most part, inherited. Actually, having allergy symptoms is part inheritance and part exposure under the right circumstances. You have a greater chance of developing an allergy if it runs in the family. Some patients, however, are adopted and have no knowledge of their birth parents' medical histories. Other patients have no knowledge because of divorce or separation from one of the parents, or the early death of one of the parents, with no available history of that part of the family, leaving the allergist guessing as to whether the patient might have inherited allergic tendencies.

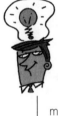

Bet You Didn't Know

A number of years ago, a researcher was able to take a strain of nonallergic mice, and then expose them to allergens plus certain external environmental conditions. This created allergies in these animals.

Where Do You Live and Work?

Equally important as your family history is the environment in which you live and work. For example, you may be exposed to chemicals in your daily life that add to your allergy problem or that work on the immune system to change its responses. Depending on the age of your home or the condition of your heating and air conditioning systems, you may be exposed to mold or other allergens during your daily activities.

How old and in what condition is your floor covering? Do you have any pets in your house or do you come into contact with pets during your daily activities? What kind of pillow do you sleep on? Is it filled with feathers or synthetic material? What do you have hanging on the walls? What else is in the room, and how frequently and thoroughly are these items cleaned? Do you sleep with open or closed windows at night?

Your allergist will also be interested in your personal habits such as drinking, smoking, and the use of herbs, home remedies, and/or recreational drugs. Alcohol not only has an adverse effect on the liver and other parts of the body, it also acts as an agent that can release histamine, which may cause allergylike symptoms such as sneezing, wheezing, and itchy eyes. Likewise, cigarette smoking can be associated with symptoms of cough, mucus in the throat, and shortness of breath. These symptoms may still prevail even if you have already kicked this nasty habit a while ago. You may think these symptoms reflect an allergy problem; your allergist, however, may be suspicious of a lung problem called chronic obstructed pulmonary disease (COPD).

Collectively, all the answers to your allergist's questions provide important information your allergist needs in order to make an informed diagnosis that identifies the hidden causes for your complaint, and separates true allergies from other problems which are nonallergic in nature.

Let's Get Physical

After establishing a medical history, your allergist may proceed with a physical examination. The examination of a patient is not unlike the act of looking at a painting. First, the allergist looks at the patient as a whole, and then he or she concentrates on the individual parts. Maintaining good eye contact with the patient, watching, and carefully listening to the patient are signs of a good diagnostician, not the least because a patient's body language and appearances can be as informative as the patient's medical history.

An initial physical examination is conducted with emphasis on areas that relate to the patient's symptoms or complaints. Thorough examination of the head and neck—including ears, nostrils, throat, and eyes—are usually first. In the neck the allergist feels for normal lymph nodes and thyroid. Next, he or she examines the shape of the chest and listens to breathing patterns and heartbeat, followed by a close look at the skin for rashes or skin changes, especially if the patient complains of hives or itching. An initial exam also includes taking the patient's blood pressure and pulse. The remainder of the physical examination typically is related to the history that has been taken by the allergist as well as the allergist's suspicions. For example, depending on the patient's symptoms, the allergist may perform a complete examination, which may include examination of the patient's joints, looking at the eyes with a special instrument to check for any abnormality, feeling the jaw to see if the headaches may be related to tempero mandibular joint (TMJ) pathology, or feeling the patient's abdomen for any enlarged organs or hernias. This history and physical examination will lead to a list of possible medical problems. This list is called a differential diagnosis.

The final diagnosis is a result of the history and the physical findings related to a differential diagnosis, which is a list of possible medical problems that could explain the symptoms.

Now that the allergist has some ideas of what might be the real cause of your symptoms, the next step would be some type of testing. Medical and allergy tests are used to verify or eliminate some of those things on the list of possible causes (differential diagnosis). In the next chapter, skin tests, blood tests, and challenges with certain allergens and/or foods will be discussed in detail.

The Least You Need to Know

♦ An allergist is a qualified medical specialist with many years of training.

♦ An accurate history is the first and most important step in diagnosing food (or other) allergies, and is a key part of your first visit to your allergist.

♦ The scope of the initial physical exam is related to the patient's medical history as well as the allergist's suspicions.

Chapter 8

Testing ... One, Two, Three

In This Chapter

- ◆ Learn which allergy tests are best for you
- ◆ Note what influences the outcome of allergy tests
- ◆ Find out how to eliminate offending foods from your diet
- ◆ Find out which allergy tests you should avoid

If your doctor suspects you have allergies, he or she can use any of a number of testing methods to identify the rogue allergen that is causing you discomfort. Testing methods include skin tests, blood tests, elimination diets, and oral challenges, all of which provide good information but are not always 100 percent accurate, and thus require that the allergist consult the patient's medical history (see previous chapter) to ensure the test results agree with it. If you want to learn more about these and other, more unconventional testing methods, this chapter is for you.

Getting Under Your Skin

Skin tests, which can be used in infants, children, and adults, are designed to measure sensitivity to specific food allergens by getting those allergens more or less, as the name implies, under your skin. These tests are based on the fact that people with allergies have excess amounts of IgE that has been programmed to recognize specific allergens. When the allergen comes in contact with the IgE antibodies, a reaction occurs that results in a chemical fallout, which in turn leaves its mark on the skin. (For more details on IgE-mediated reactions, see Chapter 2.)

Conventional allergists distinguish between two types of skin tests: *skin-prick* or *prick-puncture tests* and *intradermal tests*. The difference between the two is the degree to which they get a suspected allergen under your skin.

Med Meaning

Skin-prick or **prick-puncture tests** involve pricking or scratching the surface of the skin with a drop of the suspected allergen. In the case of **intradermal tests**, the suspected allergen is injected under the first few layers of skin with a syringe and a very fine needle.

Med Meaning

A **wheal** is a tiny swelling in the skin where the fluid leaks out of the blood vessels into the tissue. A **flare** is the red area surrounding this wheal, and occurs because the blood vessels have dilated.

Skin tests are usually done on the patient's forearms or back, with multiple allergens tested at once. For each test, your allergist creates a solution that contains an extract of a suspected allergy-producing substance—called an *allergen*—such as food extracts, pollen, dust mites, and so on.

In the case of prick-puncture tests, your allergist places a drop of each solution on the alcohol-cleaned skin, and then carefully pricks the surface of the skin through the allergy solution with a needlelike device to get some solution under the skin. (The prick isn't deep enough to cause any bleeding; it just lifts the skin surface.) After about 15 minutes, the area is carefully blotted dry and examined for *wheals* (swelling) and *flares* (redness). If the patient is sensitive to a specific allergen, the area to which it was applied will become red and form hives, each of varying size, indicating that the patient has a reaction to that particular substance. A variation of the prick-puncture test called the *scratch test* involves scratching the skin first and then applying a drop of the suspected allergen extract. However, prick-puncture tests are now considered to be more accurate than the scratch technique.

If the results of a skin-prick test are inconclusive, your allergist may conduct an *intradermal test*, which involves injecting a tiny amount of the suspected allergen into the skin with a syringe and a very fine needle. Intradermal tests are more sensitive than skin-prick procedures because they use higher concentrations of allergen extracts. For the same reason, however, they are more likely to produce adverse reactions and induce more false positive results than skin-prick tests. A false positive skin test is one in which the skin reacts with redness and swelling from the irritation of the procedure, not because of allergic reaction to the allergen put in the skin.

Measure for Measure

A very important part of skin testing is to set up a standard for measuring what is a positive response of the skin to the allergen. The standardized way of doing this is to use a planned positive and a planned negative test. This is done because each person's skin may react in an individual way. By creating a positive and negative test, doctors can accurately distinguish mere skin irritation from an allergic reaction, as well as grade the response in their testing.

To that end, the solution in which the allergen is diluted, also known as a *diluent*, is used to produce a negative test result at one prick site. A histamine solution is used to produce a true allergic reaction at another prick site. These two reactions are noted, and then all other skin tests on that patient are compared to the planned negative and positive tests.

One way to ensure the reaction is measured in a standardized way is to record the observation 15 to 20 minutes after performing the test. The actual size of each reaction is measured with a millimeter ruler.

Med Meaning

A **diluent** is the fluid in which an allergen or antigen is diluted. In the case of allergens, the diluent keeps the allergen in solution form and protects it from deteriorating, changing, or becoming contaminated. In the case of antigens, the diluent keeps the antigen fresh and pure for a given period of time.

The method of interpreting the skin tests varies with the technician and/or doctor who is reading them. Basically, each individual skin test reaction is measured with a millimeter ruler in two directions—from top to bottom and from side to side. The planned positive reactions using histamine and the planned negative reactions using diluent are recorded the same way. This creates a yardstick from negative, the diluent reaction, to positive, which is the histamine reaction. Obviously, these measurements of the foods or inhalants will not exactly match the histamine or diluent skin reaction. Here is where interpretation comes in. If the food or inhalant reaction is equal to or larger than the histamine, the reaction is said to be positive; if the skin reaction is equal to or smaller than the diluent, the reaction is read as negative. If the reaction is more than the diluent and less than the histamine, it becomes an interpretation of the observer. Other testers use a scale of 1+ up to 4+, based on a set of criteria as to the size and shape of the reaction. In general, skin testing is not an exact science; doctors use it mostly as an additional testing method to give information about possible causes of the symptoms.

When all is said and done, the allergist should take time to go over the results of the skin test procedure carefully and explain to you why certain allergens or foods were chosen for the testing.

Veritable Variables

Many factors can affect the outcome of a skin test. These factors include the following:

- **The test site on the body.** For example, the middle and upper back are more reactive than the lower back; the back is more reactive than the forearm; the area of the arm just below the bend of the elbow is more reactive than the area near the wrist. A more reactive site may also mean that it is more uncomfortable for the patient. Even though the arms are less reactive than the back, the testing is still a comparison of the allergen reaction to the histamine reaction in the same area.

- **The patient's age.** Skin testing on infants and the elderly can be positive, but the skin reaction will be smaller. Although there is no difference in the skin reactivity between men and women, women show the weakest histamine reaction during the first day of their menstrual cycle.

- **The season of the year.** In patients allergic to pollen, the skin reaction to testing is increased during and just after the pollen season. In these same patients, the size of the reaction decreases at the end of the pollen season, and remains low until the beginning of the next pollen season.

- **Existing medical conditions.** Patients on chronic hemodialysis or with eczema, cancer, or diabetes mellitus will have decreased reactions to histamine and to allergens. Also, patients who have had a systemic anaphylactic reaction should not be tested for at least two weeks after the reaction is over.

- **Certain medications.** Antihistamines may skew the outcome of a skin test by suppressing the natural response of the patient's immune system. Depending on the strength of the antihistamine, you may have to discontinue medication anywhere from 24 hours to 60 days for accurate test results. Ketotifen, tricyclic antidepressants, and antinausea agents, as well as some of the medicines used to treat asthma, can also have an effect on these results.

Skulls and Bones

Beta blockers used in treating blood pressure, headaches, and glaucoma can markedly increase the skin response to testing. Their use may lead to serious systemic anaphylaxis in the allergic patient when challenged with the allergen in the skin test. It is recommended that patients taking beta blockers not be skin tested or receive antigen injection therapy for fear of this kind of reaction.

Don't Bet Your Life on It

Allergy skin tests are cheap and easy to do. However, the predictive value of these types of tests varies depending on the patient's allergy history. For example, it is not uncommon for patients with a strong history of food allergies to have negative skin tests or weakly positive skin tests to specific foods that they know cause problems. In general, up to 50 percent of sensitive allergy patients will have a false negative reaction. Up to 15 percent of patients with low sensitivity to the allergen will have a false negative reaction.

The patient with a history of food reactions and with eczema should be tested for any information the test can provide. Positive skin tests to a food allergen indicate the possibility that the food is responsible for symptoms. However, it may also mean that despite the high levels of IgE antibodies, the person has developed a tolerance to that food and can now eat or drink it without creating a problem, as is the case with a cow's milk allergy that can occur in infancy but gradually disappear as the infant grows older. The elevated levels of IgE antibodies developed specifically in reaction to the milk allergen, however, remain in the patient's system. In this case, another testing method, called the *elimination challenge diet* (discussed later in this chapter), could provide a more accurate answer to the question.

> **CAUTION**
>
> **Skulls and Bones**
>
> Patients with a history of life-threatening reactions when exposed to a certain food or inhalant should not be tested with those particular allergens, because there is an increased chance of systemic anaphylactic reaction to the foods. However, this does not mean that doctors cannot use skin tests to test for other allergens. Intradermal tests are very effective in looking for inhalant allergies.

Seeing Red

The purpose of skin tests, when appropriate, is to gather information. The individual allergist will then interpret the accuracy and value of the information based on the type of allergy problem. If this information is not satisfactory to the allergist, he or she will consider additional tests. Depending on the results of the skin test, these additional tests may take the form of food challenges (discussed in the following section) or blood tests.

Like skin tests, blood tests are designed to measure the allergen-specific IgE levels. However, because blood tests are more expensive than skin tests without being significantly more accurate, they are only used when skin testing can be dangerous or impractical because the patient is taking antihistamines or suffers from severe skin conditions such as eczema or *dermatographism* (a condition in which the skin reacts to everything).

The most common blood test is called *radioallergosorbent test* (RAST). For this test, a sample of blood is added to the suspected allergen, and IgE activity is identified by radioactive anti-IgE antibodies. While a positive result shows the patient is sensitized to the particular allergen, it does not prove that the allergen is the cause of the symptoms.

Eliminating the Usual Suspects

The final test is to become aware of what happens when the patient is exposed to the suspected allergen. For example, if every time you eat shrimp you break out in hives, it stands to reason that you are allergic to shrimp. However, there is also a chance that you are allergic to other crustacean shellfish. The same principle applies to other foods and inhalants.

> **Timely Tip**
>
> One accurate way to gather food intelligence is to keep a food log. Note daily each item you eat, and then see if there is any relation to the onset of symptoms.

Another approach is to actively observe the effect of individual foods on the patient. If you want to put your finger on the food or group of foods that triggers your allergic reactions, ask your allergist to take a close look at your diet or food log and the results of your allergy tests, and then go through a so-called elimination challenge diet, following these steps:

1. Eliminate the suspected offending food, including other foods in the same food group, from your diet for at least two weeks. Some patients note an improvement in the symptoms just by doing that.

2. Add each of the eliminated foods from your original diet to your current diet, one food at a time at three-day intervals, and notice with which food item the symptoms return.

3. Repeat this process three times to ensure you have identified the proper food or foods.

4. Eliminate the offending food or foods from your diet for good.

> **Timely Tip**
>
> Patients and nursing mothers who are totally successful with elimination diets must pay attention to their nutrition. The nutrients that could be affected are calcium, protein, vitamins, and minerals.

A variation of this type of elimination diet is the *elemental diet*. In this diet, foods are broken down into small molecules. The diet is consumed in liquid form. During the initial two weeks, the diet is limited to this liquid food. Again, the next step is to add back foods, one at a time, at three-day intervals. The major drawback is that the food in this diet tastes dreadful, and it is very expensive. This type of procedure should be done with your doctor's supervision.

You can experiment with different members of a food group to see if you can tolerate one member of the group but not another. The best example of this is peanuts and other legumes. Some patients are allergic to peanuts, but not to other members of the legume group, such as soy.

What are the odds that if you are allergic to one food in a food group, you will be allergic to another food in the same group?

- If you are allergic to peanuts, you have a 5 percent risk of having an allergic reaction to other legumes such as peas, lentils, or beans.

- If you are allergic to a tree nut (like a walnut), you have a 37 percent chance of having a reaction to other tree nuts (like brazil, cashew, or hazelnut).

- If you are allergic to salmon, there is a 50 percent chance of your having a reaction to other fish (like swordfish or sole).

- If you are allergic to shrimp, there is a 75 percent chance you would have a reaction to other crustaceans (like crab and lobster).

- If you are allergic to a grain like wheat, you have a 20 percent chance of being allergic to other grains (like barley and rye).

- If you are allergic to cow's milk, there is a 10 percent chance you would have a reaction to beef (like hamburger) and a 92 percent chance you would have a reaction to goat's milk.

- If you are allergic to pollen (like birch and ragweed), there is a 55 percent chance you will have a reaction to fruits and vegetables (like apples, peaches, and honeydew).

- If you are allergic to melon (cantaloupe), there is a 92 percent chance that you will react to avocado, watermelon, and bananas.

- If you are allergic to peaches, there is a 55 percent chance you will react to plums, pears, apples, and cherries.

- If you are allergic to latex, there is a 35 percent chance you will react to kiwi, bananas, and avocados.

- If you are allergic to fruits (banana, kiwi, and avocados), you have an 11 percent chance of being allergic to latex.

Taking on Food Challenges

There are two additional testing methods that have been designed for use within a medical setting: "open" or "single-blind" challenge and "double-blind" challenge testing.

The "Open" Challenge

In "open" challenge testing, the food being tested is known or "open" to the patient and the allergist. In this type of challenge, the patient must eliminate all foods of the suspected food group from the diet for at least two weeks prior to the test. In addition, the patient should avoid using antihistamines or other medications that might cloud the test results.

The challenge is then started as a so-called single-blind study, meaning your allergist is one step ahead of the patient in this game. In the doctor's office, the patient is given increasingly concentrated amounts of the specific food, disguised in lyophilized or powdered form in a gelatin capsule that the patient swallows whole. The dose is doubled every 15 to 60 minutes until it reaches a dose of 10 grams of this food. Throughout this period, as more and more of the food is administered, the patient is closely observed for any reactions. If the reaction is negative, then the patient is given the food in an open feeding to observe any reactions.

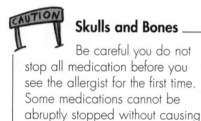

Skulls and Bones

Be careful you do not stop all medication before you see the allergist for the first time. Some medications cannot be abruptly stopped without causing harm to the patient.

Because the patient is "consuming" increasingly concentrated amounts of the offending food, it is mandatory that this type of testing be done in the doctor's office; in case of a serious allergic reaction, the doctor and the proper emergency equipment are readily available.

The "Double-Blind" Challenge

The double-blind placebo-controlled food challenge, or "double-blind" challenge for short, is the only scientifically validated test to learn if a certain food (or drug) is causing allergic problems.

Similar to the "open" challenge, the patient is kept off the suspected food group and is instructed not to take antihistamines or other medications. The challenge is administered to the patient on an empty stomach. In this form of testing, neither the patient nor the physician knows whether the administered gelatin capsule contains the suspected food allergen or a placebo (with no allergen). That is why this is called a *double-blind study*. The patient receives both placebo and suspected food during the test.

Food challenge tests are typically time-consuming and are mostly used for research purposes, or when there is doubt that a food is triggering a patient's allergic reaction.

Get Thee to a Laboratory

There are still other tests for food allergies. Some of these are done in research laboratories, and provide information about the amount of histamine released from mast cells when challenged by individual foods. The test results provide reliable information, but are not commonly available in an allergist's office.

These tests include the following:

♦ **BHR (Basophil Histamine Release) assay.** In this test the cells are challenged directly by the suspected allergen, to see if the basophil cells release histamine. Next, it is used to see if the addition of new drugs will interfere with this reaction. This test can be used in research, but is of little value in diagnosing food allergies in a person.

♦ **IMCHR (Intestinal Mast Cell Histamine Release).** In this test, the mast cells, another form of basophil, are obtained from the lining of the intestinal tract. Once again, the same challenge is done in a test tube to get the same type of information.

♦ **IPEC (Intragastral Provocation under Endoscopy).** In this test, the food is placed on the lining of the patient's stomach or other parts of the gastrointestinal tract. The reaction is observed through an endoscope and recorded on film to study later. This is almost like a skin test, but done on the gut.

♦ **Intestinal biopsy after allergen elimination and feeding.** In this type of test, a sample of intestinal tissue is taken, after directly exposing that part of the gut to the suspected food. This is a surgical procedure, done strictly as research, to learn how the body reacts. Obviously, it would be impractical to do as a screening test, since it needs very specialized lab and surgical equipment, as well as people experienced in the procedure. As surgical procedures, these carry all the possible complications of surgery. Further, they have no benefit as screening procedures at present.

All of these tests are strictly done for research purposes.

The Least You Need to Know

♦ Skin-prick and blood tests are designed to measure IgE sensitization in patients.

♦ Helpful information comes from food diary observation.

♦ Food challenge tests give the most accurate information about food allergies.

Chapter 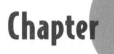9

Show Me the Meds

In This Chapter

- ◆ Discover what medications provide relief from allergic reactions
- ◆ Understand how antihistamines work
- ◆ Learn about the good and bad effects of antihistamines
- ◆ Find out what new allergy treatments are on the horizon

Planning allergy-safe meals requires a lot of discipline; avoiding the foods that bother you can be a challenge, too. The person with food allergies may make an honest try at avoidance, but nevertheless still accidentally consume or come in contact with the offending food. Depending on the patient, the result of this accidental encounter can be anywhere from uncomfortable to fatal. When adverse results ensue, what can be done about them? What magic help does medical science offer?

This chapter helps you sort through your treatment options.

Ease My Sneeze

A talented patient/poet who prefers to remain anonymous wrote the following to describe her allergy problems:

Hey, Doc,
My nose is stuffed,
My head is full;
I sneeze a lot,
I need a pill.
Am I allergic to the dust?
Or is it ragweed I can't trust?

Yes, this lady needs a pill; but there are so many different ones in so many different categories, and therefore so many choices. Yet all have one thing in common: They're all designed to block the effects of the chemical that is responsible for your allergic symptoms—histamine.

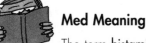

Med Meaning

The term **histamine** comes from the words *hist*, meaning "related to tissue," and *amine*, which is the tissue's chemical structure.

As you learned in Chapter 2, histamine is an important mediator released by mast cells during Type I immune system responses and the inflammatory response which can follow. Remember, immune system responses and inflammation can be good things. They are your body's defense against harmful and, in the case of food allergies, frequently not-so-harmful substances that find a way into your body.

The symptoms that histamine release produces depend on the end organ affected, and include mucus secretion, nitrous oxide formation, and cell contraction; this in turn leads to increased permeability or breakdown of blood vessels, gastric acid secretion, and contraction of muscles in our bronchial tubes. If the skin were the end organ, the symptoms would be itching, swelling, welts, or hives. If the end organ were the respiratory system, the symptoms would be sneezing, nasal congestion, watery nose, or even wheezing and shortness of breath if the lungs were involved.

Med Meaning

The term **receptor** comes from the French word *recevoir*, meaning "to receive." A receptor on a cell is a protein molecule on the cell surface or within the cell that binds to a drug, hormone, allergen, or neurotransmitter.

Antihistamines are designed to block the effects of histamine. They work by binding to *receptors* on the mast cells or basophils, thus reducing histamine release and the natural next steps that can lead to allergy symptoms. Some people refer to these as "competitive inhibitors." Antihistamines can be used to reduce food allergy symptoms as well as reduce stomach acid in patients with ulcers or acid reflux problems. Those that are effective on the stomach are called *H2 receptor inhibitors*; these act to reduce the amount of acid production in the stomach.

The antihistamines you may use for symptoms of food allergies are labeled according to the receptor site they will most commonly bind to.

♦ H1 receptors can be found in areas of skin, nose, eyes, throat, lungs, and so on. These are areas people usually associate with allergies.

♦ H2 receptors are found in the gut and are related to acid production.

♦ H3 receptors appear to help control the amount of histamine produced. This also works in parts of the nervous system around blood vessels. H3 receptors can dilate blood vessels in the brain and decrease certain chemical release in the airways controlled by the vagus nerve. (For more details on the vagus nerve, see Chapter 5.)

H3 receptors may also be a defense mechanism against constriction of our lungs. This is still to be proven. In still other areas, they cause blood platelets to stick together.

Antihistamines Old and New

The first antihistamines that were perfected were those that attach to H1 type receptors. They are also referred to as first-generation antihistamines, because another group was developed from these chemicals at a later time and called—you guessed it— second-generation antihistamines.

Let's look at this class of antihistamines more closely.

A Few Unpronounceables

First-generation agents are divided into groups according to their chemical structures. They include …

♦ **Ethanolamine.** Benedryl, Dramamine, Tavist.

♦ **Alkylamines.** Chlortrimeton, Dimetane, Drixoral, Polaramine, Actifed, Triaminic, Rynatan.

♦ **Ethylenediamines.** Pyrobenzamine, Vasocon A.

♦ **Piperazines.** Atarax, Bonine, Antivert, Marezine.

♦ **Phenothiazines.** Phenergan, Tacaryl, Temeril.

♦ **Piperidines.** Periactin, Optamine, Trinalin.

Bet You Didn't Know _____

Some people with food allergies also have inhalant allergies; in fact, one may increase the other. Taking an antihistamine before an allergic reaction gives the medication more time to get a head start. Begin your antihistamine before you are exposed to known allergens, or before the pollen season starts.

Because these medications are structurally different, they do have different uses and side effects. Some of them cause drowsiness to a greater or lesser extent, while others are more effective for itching or hives. Another group is very effective for nausea or vomiting.

First-generation antihistamines actually compete for the histamine-receptor-binding site on the cell. If the antihistamine gets there first (before the histamine) and attaches, then the histamine is prevented from attaching to the cell and the histamine response is blocked.

Relief Is Just a Swallow Away

Antihistamines are rapidly absorbed from the stomach or blood. They can give symptom relief in thirty minutes, and are removed by liver enzymes.

First-generation antihistamines cross from the blood into the central nervous system, breast milk, and the placenta. Going into the central nervous system can cause drowsiness, as a result of this crossover into the central nervous system.

Antihistamines work by binding the H1 receptor sites, so that the histamine cannot dock and react. However, this is an active, ongoing process, because the antihistamines are being broken down constantly by the cells in the immune system. This opens up the binding site to once again be available to histamine. Whether histamine or antihistamine will bind to an available receptor site ultimately depends on the amount of each in the bloodstream. If the amount of antihistamine drops, then there is more chance for histamine to move in and bind to the receptor. In other words, you need lots of troops to outnumber the enemy.

Timely Tip _____

Patients need to use their antihistamine on a regular schedule to maintain enough in the bloodstream to give maximal therapeutic value.

From First to Second

First-generation antihistamines work well, but have some problems. They need to be taken regularly to maintain a high blood level; they cross the blood-brain barrier and create drowsiness; and they have a cholinergic effect on other organs, which means that the medication reacts on certain nerve fibers and their neurotransmitters, to cause drying of certain membranes and/or spasm in the urinary bladder, thus creating problems urinating.

Med Meaning _____

Blood-brain barrier is a term used to describe the lining capillaries of the central nervous system. Any medication that crosses the blood-brain barrier has an effect on the function of the central nervous system. In the case of antihistamines, the effects are to cause drowsiness and prevent nausea. A **neurotransmitter** is a specific chemical agent released by nerve cells. This chemical crosses a gap to stimulate or inhibit another nerve cell.

In response to this drawback, researchers developed so-called second-generation, non-sedating antihistamines, which differ from first-generation antihistamines in terms of their chemical structure as well as their properties. For example, second-generation antihistamines, like first-generation antihistamines, bind to H1 receptors. Unlike their seniors, however, second-generation antihistamines release from these receptors very slowly, and are not affected by high concentrations of histamine in the circulation. Another property is that they do not easily cross the blood-brain barrier, so there is little drowsiness associated.

Second-generation antihistamines include Fexofenadine (Allegra), Loratadine (Claritin), and Cetirizine (Zyrtec), as well as Terfenadine (Seldane) and Astemizole (Hismanol), both of which are no longer available in the U.S. market, because of safety concerns. First-generation antihistamines work faster for immediate symptoms. Second-generation antihistamines take longer to help, but are just as effective and useful for long-term symptoms, since they do not leave the patient groggy or interfere with daily activity.

Dissolved in Fat, Fond of Water

Both first- and second-generation antihistamines are described as either lipophilic or lipophobic. A medication that has a tendency to move from the bloodstream into the tissue is called *lipophilic*, having an affinity for fats (lipids); *lipos* (Greek for "fat") and *philic* (Greek for "fond of") together mean "able to be dissolved in fat."

Medication that does not easily move into tissue and fat cells is called *lipophobic*—*phobia* comes from the Greek *phobos* meaning "fear." Medication that does not easily move into tissue with fat prefers tissue with water, such as blood vessels. These medications are also called *hydrophilic*—having a strong affinity for water.

Med Meaning _____

Lipophilic drugs prefer tissue or fat cells. They are also called *hydrophobic*. **Lipophobic** drugs prefer water, and are also called *hydrophilic*.

Sticking Things Out

Patients commonly complain that first-generation antihistamines work quickly for acute, right now symptoms, but that on the other hand, the effects of these medications are gone within four to six hours. Then patients try the second-generation, nonsedating antihistamines, but find that they don't work as fast.

The second-generation antihistamine binds more slowly, but once attached, stays in place for a longer period of time.

Patients using Allegra or Claritin must understand that it can take up to two or three days for them to act in their most forceful way. In either case, it's important to continue the antihistamine on a regular routine as long as you are exposed to the allergen or are recovering from an allergic reaction.

There are other medications that have antihistamine properties. Tricyclic antidepressants such as Doxepin are also antihistamines. These drugs have a very high attraction for H1 receptors, and are used for patients with chronic hives.

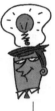

> **Bet You Didn't Know** _____
>
> People who are in a car accident and are taking antihistamines can be booked under DUI (driving under the influence) charges in most states.

> **Skulls and Bones** _____
>
> Alcohol increases the severity of the side effects of most medications. In the case of antihistamines, it will increase drowsiness and will slow the reaction time. A little bit of alcohol plus antihistamine is very dangerous in driving a vehicle or in working with heavy machinery. In fact, it would be unwise to take a test or exam under those conditions, because the mind is dulled. (Tell that to the SAT board.)

The Right Stuff

Now that you understand all of the different types of antihistamines, it's important to know which ones to use and when to use them.

- **Common allergy symptoms.** Both first- and second-generation antihistamines are equally good for most common allergy symptoms such as runny nose, itchy, watery eyes, and sneezing, as well as eczema, hives, and general allergic reactions.

- **Allergy-induced skin disorders.** Hydroxyzine (Atarax) and Diphenhydramine (Benedryl) are very effective in relieving the symptoms of allergic skin disorders such as hives and eczema. These antihistamines give greater anti-itching relief and more sedation. Cyproheptadine (Periactin) is also very effective for chronic hives and severe itching of chicken pox.

♦ **Antihistamines in asthmatic patients.** The use of antihistamines in asthma has been a controversial problem for many years. The worry was that some antihistamines have a drying effect on tissues of the lungs, which could make the asthma worse. We have learned that allergies can be a trigger to start an asthma reaction. Antihistamines can stop the allergic reaction, and hopefully block the allergic trigger.

Bet You Didn't Know _____

The first line of therapy for anaphylaxis is still using adrenalin or epinephrine, but antihistamines are helping in treating the allergic part of this reaction. Antihistamines can be given just after the epinephrine, but will not start to work as fast as epinephrine. The combined result is an immediate and slightly delayed help.

Safe for Baby and More

It is advisable that pregnant women take only medication that is safe for the developing baby. Long-term experience shows that two safe medications are Chlorpheneramine and Diphenhydramine. They cause no greater risk for birth defects than in pregnant women who do not take antihistamines. If possible, all medications should be avoided until after the first three months of the pregnancy.

Another place that antihistamines work is in conditions such as motion sickness, dizziness, nausea, anxiety, or insomnia. This is because the first-generation antihistamines cross the blood-brain barrier and affect the central nervous system to decrease these symptoms. Dramamine and its derivatives work best in these conditions.

Skulls and Bones _____

Antihistamines taken by a nursing mother will come through into the breast milk. Infants nursing on this breast milk may show signs of sedation or drowsiness as a side effect of the mother's antihistamine.

Safety First

The H1 antihistamines are good to use for a variety of symptoms. Unfortunately, this category of medications comes with several side effects that you should be aware of. Specific examples include slowed reaction time, drowsiness, confusion, dizziness, ringing in the ears, loss of appetite or nausea, vomiting, stomach pain, diarrhea, or constipation.

Some people experience dry mouth, blurred vision, or difficulty urinating, while others experience weight gain as a side effect. A side effect for men taking antihistamine could be impotence.

A special warning: Antihistamines will make alcohol and antianxiety medication more potent. Second-generation antihistamines have fewer side effects and cause less drowsiness, but patients sometimes report side or flank area pain, a sense of being nervous, or interference with sleep.

Some of these medications, including Hisminol and Seldane, have been prohibited for sale or use in the United States, because of possible side effects related to the heart. The problems concerned the high concentration of those particular antihistamines that accumulated in the bloodstream.

Listen to Your Stomach

H2 receptors are found in the stomach lining where they are ready to bind to H2 receptor antagonists (H2 antihistamines). Their main use is to decrease problems with gastric acids.

Like H1 antihistamines, H2 antihistamines act by competing for the receptor site against histamine. However, H2 antihistamines are less lipophilic, so they stay in the secretions. These drugs—Zantac, Pepcid, and Axid—work best in the stomach to decrease acid. They are proven not to be very effective against other allergy problems.

Antihistamines have a close structural resemblance to histamine because most of them were derived from the histamine molecule. For the most part, histamine is more attracted to H1 receptors.

These H2 antihistamines were developed specifically to control gastric acidity. In turn, they do not work well for general allergy problems, such as nasal and eye symptoms, but they have been used along with H1 antihistamines to control chronic hives of unknown cause.

H2 antihistamines do have a downside. Some interact with other medications by slowing down the ability of the liver to remove them. As a result, these other medications—like heart and pain medications, cortisone, theophyllin used for asthma, and coumadin—will increase in the blood, because the liver cannot remove them.

Antagonists at Grand Central

H3 receptor antagonists are found in the brain. Receptor antagonists is another term for antihistamines, and is more descriptive of how they work. They tie up the receptor on the cell, so that the histamine cannot attach to the cell and start the allergic reaction.

In 1983, it was discovered that histamine in the brain binds to these H3 type receptors and may result in a decreased production of histamine in the central nervous system.

The process literally turns itself off. (Talk about automation!) The name used for this is negative feedback. H1 and H2 antihistamines do not stop this process.

> **Skulls and Bones**
>
> Taking antihistamines before exposure to foods that cause known severe reactions does not prevent anaphylactic or possibly fatal reactions.

Small Steps, Small Solutions

One medication available for symptoms produced by food allergies is oral Cromolyn Sodium, called *Gastrocrome*. This medication works by preventing the breakdown of mast cells and is described as being a mast cell stabilizer. The actual amount of improvement using this medication is variable. The way it works is that it helps to decrease the breakdown of mast cells in the gastrointestinal tract.

In our definition of food hypersensitivity, the reaction involves IgE attaching to the mast cell. The allergen hooks on to the IgE, which in turn destabilizes the mast cell membrane. This destabilization results in histamine and chemical mediators being released into the circulation.

The symptoms produced depend on the end organ affected. If the skin were the end organ, the symptoms would be itching, swelling, welts, or hives. If the end organ were the respiratory system, the symptoms would be sneezing, nasal congestion, watery nose, or even wheezing and shortness of breath, if the lungs were involved. Therapy for asthmalike symptoms is the same as treating any acute asthma problem.

Cromolyn Sodium stabilizes the mast cell; therefore it should be taken before the patient eats and before the allergic food gets into the system. The advised method is to use this medication 4 times a day, about 30 to 40 minutes before eating. It works best if taken on an empty stomach.

Patients who have adhered to this regimen say it provides mild to moderate help, but that they must be very vigilant, almost compulsive, to take the medication as suggested. It does not make them symptom-free or allow them an unrestricted diet. It does seem to decrease the allergic reaction, so that they can extend their diet to include more foods, but still in small amounts.

Med Miracles?

Some antihistamines work best after the allergic reaction occurs. Examples of helpful antihistamines are Benedryl and Chlortrimeton, as well as other over-the-counter products.

Nonsedating second-generation antihistamines such as Allegra and Claritin work well, but will take longer to give maximum results.

All of these antihistamines work best for treating symptoms such as hives, itching, swelling, and nasal congestion and/or sneezing. Some patients have tried taking these antihistamines before knowingly eating the offending foods. This does not prevent the allergic reaction from occurring, but it may, in the opinion of many patients, decrease the severity of the allergic reaction and make the symptoms more bearable.

Take Your Meds

Important medications are those that control the itching that can result from food allergies. Usually antihistamines are used for relief. Some are more effective than others (such as the Hydroxyzine group and Benadryl).

Some of these antihistamines cause more drowsiness, which is fine at night but a real problem during the day. But not to worry; with the availability of second-generation, nonsedating antihistamines, this problem can be removed. One thing you should understand about this class of antihistamines is that they may take two to three days before they are really effective. Then the medication should be continued on a regular basis. It is most important to control the itch.

Skin infection is a common complication of atopic dermatitis, which may have been made worse by food allergies. The infection must be treated properly. The best way to treat the infection is with the appropriate antibiotic taken by mouth. Occasionally, antibiotic creams will be suggested for minor skin infections, or to use along with antibiotics taken by mouth.

Bet You Didn't Know

Antihistamines are among the top four categories of pharmaceutical products sold, and account for billions of dollars spent annually. Seniors are among the prime purchasers of these drugs.

Your physician should prescribe the particular antibiotic you use. Topical antibiotics, those applied to the skin, have limited usefulness. In fact, some will sensitize the skin and make the eczema worse. In some cases, the chemical vehicle used with corticosteroid creams are the sensitizing agent that makes the situation worse.

Lives at Stake

Epinephrine or adrenaline is a medication that is used to treat a life-threatening allergic reaction. If you accidentally eat a food you are allergic to and develop a severe anaphylactic reaction, this medication is your lifesaver. It is given by injection. One prescription name of this is Anakit; another, which is an auto-injector, is called EpiPen.

The EpiPen comes as an adult dose and as EpiPen Junior, which is a dose for children. In a severe allergic reaction there can be widening or dilation of blood vessels that leads to a drop in blood pressure, shock, and possible stopping of the heart and/or lungs. Adrenaline works by making the blood vessels contract. Antihistamines can be given at the same time, but are not a substitute for adrenaline.

> **CAUTION**
>
> **Skulls and Bones**
>
> Patients on ACE inhibitors or beta-blocking medication are resistant to the effects of adrenaline. If these people have an anaphylactic reaction, adrenaline is not indicated and may even make the reaction more severe. The emergency room physician or other health-care giver should have Glucagon available.

Deadly Delayed Reactions

Delayed food allergic reactions can occur up to six to eight hours after exposure to the allergen. Symptoms of this type of reaction are similar to those that can occur within a few minutes to 30 minutes after the initial exposure.

They include itching, swelling, nausea, stomach pain, hoarseness, feeling a lump in the throat, sneezing, runny nose, weakness, warmth, sense of apprehension or dread, disorientation, or loss of bodily functions. Get help!

If you have severe food allergies, you should consider having a Medic Alert bracelet, and emergency medical service numbers (such as 911) should be within reach in your living area.

Prednisone is indicated to stop allergic reactions that are not improving or coming under control with antihistamines. A second situation in which to use this medication is to prevent a delayed allergic reaction or delayed anaphylactic reaction. A delayed reaction is one that happens 8 to 12 hours after an immediate first allergic reaction. This means an allergic reaction can happen in two stages. The first, immediately after exposure to the allergen, and again, 8 to 12 hours later.

The use of cortisone at the correct times is important and can even be a lifesaver. This is especially true when treating anaphylactic or delayed reactions in severe, systemic food allergy reactions. The correct, safe dose of any medication is dependent on how the body reacts to the medication and how easily the body can cleanse itself of the breakdown products of that medication. A normally functioning liver and kidneys are vital for this to work correctly.

Therefore, some medicines, such as cortisone, depend on the liver to break them down for removal from the circulation. The process that occurs within the liver depends on certain natural enzymes. These enzymes can be blocked by some medications, so that the process cannot go on. Turning off the process of removal causes a gradual, progressive increase in the amount of medication in the circulation. This increased amount can reach harmful or toxic levels. Another, more common, example of liver toxicity occurs in patients with chronic liver disease, such as hepatitis or cirrhosis. Awareness of problems of kidney or liver failure means the patient should take lower doses to accomplish the same benefit without bad side effects. In these cases, the attending doctor will make the necessary adjustments in dosage. It does not mean you cannot take the medication when it is needed. It does mean it must be taken in proper amounts. The other side of this is in cases where a patient seems to react as if they have taken too large a dose; the doctor should make sure there no unrecognized liver or kidney problems.

Med Meaning

Cortisone could be defined as a medication which acts to decrease inflammation. **Hepatitis** refers to the inflammation of the liver due to viral infections or toxic agents. The origin of the word is from the Greek *kirrhos*, meaning "yellow," plus *osis*, meaning "condition." **Cirrhosis** is end-stage liver disease with widespread damage to the cells, nodules, and scarring. This is associated with failure of liver function and blockage of blood flow to the liver.

The Future of Allergy Research

Are patients happy with what present-day medical science provides as food allergy treatments? Not exactly. Are today's food allergy solutions as good as it gets? So far, yes. Can't we do better? We're trying. So what does the future hold for potential new food allergy solutions? Even while you are reading this, researchers are hard at work finding new pathways in food allergy treatment.

Several new ideas and theories on how to handle food allergies loom on the horizon. Some researchers at major medical facilities would like to alter the genes of the specific food that controls the protein content. Others are thinking in terms of removing entirely the offending allergenic protein from the food. A third group argues to simply modify the allergenic protein itself.

Skulls and Bones

There is more than one protein in a specific food that causes the allergic reaction. Removing, modifying, or suppressing the protein may wind up killing the plant.

If you can't change the food, then changing the allergic person's reaction to food is one direction researchers are looking into. Suggestions have included gastric mucosa, stomach lining, and vaccines to change the reaction of the lining of the intestinal tract. Still another approach is immune therapy that would change the level of mediators in the immune system.

Seriously, What's Brewing?

Some researchers have gone past the maybe and could be stages. These different groups are trying to find ways to remove the danger to those with severe food allergies. Here is a list of their diverse efforts:

♦ **Oral therapy.** This has been tried on animals using pollen. In this approach, large doses of pollen are given by mouth, which creates in the animals a tolerance to future exposure. This seems to work in animal experiments, but has mixed results in people. People with respiratory allergies were given large doses of pollen to swallow over a period of time. Some patients reported only slight decreases of their symptoms, while others felt no difference at all. The safety and success of this approach is questionable, and trying this approach with food has been unsuccessful.

♦ **Immune complex approach.** According to this treatment solution, using the allergen to which a patient is allergic attached to an antibody to the specific allergen is another possible treatment suggested for future use. The specific allergen-antibody combination is derived from the serum portion of the blood of other people allergic to the same allergen. This approach is very complicated to carry out; so far it has only been tried out on pollen, not on foods. Since the antigen-antibody is removed from the serum, there is little chance of transferring diseases like hepatitis or HIV. Plans are to try to apply it on food allergies in the future.

♦ **New vaccine solution.** Some researchers are trying to inject a peptide fragment that is only part of the allergic portion of the protein. Because it is not a complete protein, it will not cross-link with the IgE molecule on the mast cells. The advantage is that standard antigen injection or vaccine injection therapy could be carried out without adverse effects. Sounds good, but it is very expensive.

♦ **Mucosal vaccines.** These vaccines are theorized to increase the level of IgA and IgG. In this case, the allergen is attached to another substance, such as a chemical-treated bacteria. This makes the bacteria harmless, but the combination will increase the amount of IgA and will be nontoxic. This can create tolerance or even suppression, if given in large amounts. Once again, this has been done with inhalant allergens, but not food.

♦ **Probiotics.** This suggested method involves applying certain strains or types of lactobacilli to the gut wall. The theory is that this might improve the intestinal flora and protect the gut against pathogens or allergens. Once again, there are no reports of major success.

This Could Be the Start of Something Big

Now here are two methods that sound promising.

One method is simply called the anti-IgE method. The first thing to do is to produce anti-IgE antibodies. These antibodies will attach to the IgE and block it from working. The process decreases the overall production of IgE, since it also blocks the signal to the immune system to make more IgE. This method has been tried on humans and looks promising and safe.

Recently, another approach, called *DNA immunization*, has begun to be perfected. This DNA comes from the allergen. Once injected and picked up by the person's bloodstream, it reacts with T cells responsible for limiting the amount of IgE that is produced.

Promising work is being done and more allergens are being used. This may be the beginning of something *big*—and none too soon for the millions of food allergy sufferers seeking a better solution to their problems.

The frustration felt by so many is expressed in the following thoughts. Tacked to the doctor's office door, a desperate, anonymous poet left his allergist a note that reads:

> I woke up with a terrible cough
> I had some itchy eyes.
> I know that I don't have a cold,
> But much to my surprise,
> When I looked upon my arm
> I even saw some hives
>
> And so I come to visit you,
> My doctor tried and true.
> Please diagnose my allergies,
> 'Cause I don't have a clue.
>
> Do check out the foods I eat.
> I try new ones every day;
> I know I have reactions,
> So, now I have to pay.
>
> I know that some folks can't drink milk
> And others can't eat fish;
> Eggs and wheat cause problems too.
> Do you know what's in a knish?

Hopefully, someday we will know "what's in a knish"—and have all the answers to so many other perplexing food allergy problems as well.

The Least You Need to Know

- There are many types of antihistamines, including first- and second-generation antihistamines.

- The second-generation antihistamines are considered nonsedating.

- H2 antihistamines help control gastrointestinal problems related to stomach acid.

- Patients should be educated to the possible side effects of all medications.

- Promising new approaches to treating food allergies are on the horizon.

Part 4

The Allergic Family

Hope springs eternal, and in the case of food allergies, hoping can lead to successful coping when you follow the right guidelines. From pregnancy to birth to the older child to older adults, this section covers all members of your family's food allergy and intolerance problems, including tips for shopping for allergy-safe foods and dining out, and even includes solutions for your pets—yes, they, too, have the same adverse food reactions we humans do.

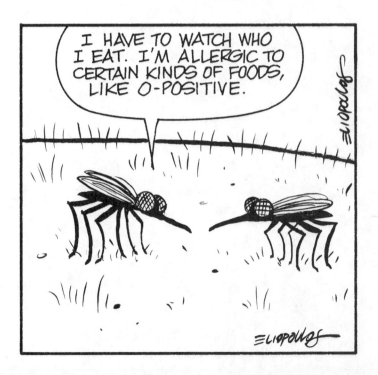

10

Preventing and Treating Food Problems in Children

In This Chapter

◆ Identifying the allergic baby

◆ Understanding the benefits of breast-feeding

◆ Feeding advice for mothers of infants

◆ Dealing with food allergies in the older child

Researchers and practicing clinician physicians estimate that from 4 to 6 percent of children under 3 years of age have allergies to certain foods. To delay, maybe prevent, or at least recognize the presence of this, you should be aware of what you as a parent or other family members can do for your infant. The symptoms of food allergies can take many forms, depending on which part of the body is affected. Most food allergic reactions are not life-threatening, but can cause annoying symptoms. The most common symptoms affecting the respiratory tract of babies and children are runny nose and itchy, red, swollen eyes. Skin symptoms include eczema and other itchy rashes; and symptoms in the intestinal tract include vomiting, diarrhea, and stomach pain. This chapter takes you through the chances of a food allergy occurring in your infant, and discusses what you can do to delay or prevent it.

It also provides information about introducing solids in your baby's diet and what you should know about food allergies in older children.

The Food Allergy Guessing Game

Wouldn't it be nice if science had a method to identify allergy-prone children at birth so parents could take appropriate steps immediately? Alas, there is no genetic marker in the case of allergies. Whether the child will develop allergies in infancy or beyond depends on so many variables ranging from family history to environmental exposure to the child's diet—it is, as doctors like to call it, multi-factorial. For example, the first factor is the specific food itself; secondly, we must weigh how strong is the family history of allergy; and last, we must also consider the environment, including smog, cigarette smoke, dust mites, infection, and diesel oil emissions.

A general rule of thumb expressed by allergy physicians is the following:

- If neither parent has allergies, there is about a 12 percent to 15 percent chance of the child developing allergies.

- If one parent has allergies such as allergic rhinitis, eczema, or asthma, there is about a 50 percent chance that the infant will have allergic tendencies.

- If both parents have allergies, most doctors say there is a risk factor as high as 60 percent to 70 percent.

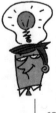

Bet You Didn't Know

As population moves from rural to urban (city) setting, there seems to be an increase in the number of allergies, possibly caused by factors in the environment.

This information refers to allergies in general. Only about 2 percent of the group will develop true food allergies.

Observation in clinical practice also has shown that there is an increased chance for the infant to have an allergy when there is a history of proven allergy in brothers, sisters, aunts, uncles, or grandparents.

Bet You Didn't Know

A more accurate method of predicting whether a child is allergy-prone is to measure the IgE level in the blood from the umbilical cord at birth. If there is an elevated level of IgE and the mother has proven allergies, then there is at least a 50 percent chance that the infant will have allergy problems. Alternatively, you could ask an allergist to do a prick-puncture skin test for specific foods such as eggs, cow's milk, and peanuts. Skin test results in infants are generally smaller skin reactions, but can be positive. These become more accurate as the child gets older and is exposed to the foods in question.

Furthermore, there is a 40 percent chance that an infant allergic to cow's milk, soy, egg, or wheat will eventually develop a tolerance to these foods.

What Are the Chances of Having a Food Allergy?

The following list provides an overview of an infant's chances to develop a food allergy:

- 6 percent of allergies occur in infants younger than 3 years of age.
- 2.5 percent of newborns have reactions to cow's milk in the first year of life.
- 80 percent of these 2.5 percent "outgrow" their allergies by 5 years of age.
- 25 percent of the remaining group will continue to have problems until they are in their twenties.
- 35 percent of newborns with cow's milk allergy will acquire other food allergies.
- 1.5 percent are allergic to eggs in early childhood (no ages given).
- 0.5 percent develop allergies to peanuts in early childhood (no ages given).
- 35 percent of patients with atopic dermatitis/eczema have food allergies involving IgE.
- 6 percent of asthma patients have wheezing caused by food allergies.
- 0.5 to 1.0 percent of children have adverse effects to food additives.
- 1.1 percent of American adults are allergic to peanuts and tree nuts.
- 2 percent of American adults have food allergies.
- 85 percent of children with food allergies are allergic to cow's milk, eggs, peanuts, fish, soy, or wheat. (Adults are mostly allergic to peanuts, tree nuts, fish, and shellfish.)

The preceding information has been adapted from *The Journal of Allergy and Clinical Immunology Primer on Allergic and Immunologic Diseases,* Volume III No. 2, Feb. 2003. The author is Hugh A. Sampson, M.D.

Recognizing Allergies

Recognizing allergies is sometimes very difficult. The parent or the patient needs to be aware not only of symptoms, but of their relationship to eating certain foods or being exposed to specific allergens in their environment. Examples are hives after eating chocolate, or sneezing when someone is cutting the grass. The following table provides an overview of symptoms in each part of the body.

Food Allergic Disorders

Area	Symptoms
Skin	Hives, tissue swelling (angioedema), rashes, flushing
Gastrointestinal	Gastrointestinal anaphylaxis with cramping, abdominal pain, vomiting, or diarrhea
Oral	An itching of the gums or lining of the mouth and/or blister-like rash on the gums
Respiratory	Acute runny nose; red, itchy, swollen eyes; wheezing
General	Anaphylaxis, shock (the most common causes are peanuts and tree nuts)

These symptoms can emerge at various times, depending on the system. Hives, swelling, or rashes usually occur within minutes of eating the foods that cause the allergic reaction. This is also true of gastrointestinal problems such as wheat, soy, or cow's milk. Chronic symptoms of runny nose and eczema may occur gradually and are ongoing, since the foods causing these symptoms are used as a basic part of the diet, like cow's milk and eggs.

Food intolerance sometimes will be mistaken for food allergies. Feeding an infant large amounts of juice or fruits may cause diarrhea. Feeding an infant red-colored juice may be mistaken for blood. Feeding the baby large amounts of cow's milk without any vegetables or meats may lead to anemia, with the baby looking pale and acting listless. (This happens because cow's milk lacks iron, which is needed to make red blood cells, so that a diet exclusively of cow's milk will not provide the iron needed.)

The most common symptoms of food allergies involve the gastrointestinal tract and the skin.

Itchy Foods and Other Culprits

Atopic dermatitis, or *eczema* as it is more commonly known, refers to an inflammation of the skin that usually occurs in persons with a (family) history of allergies. The condition frequently starts in infancy or early childhood, and decreases in severity with age. The degree of the rash's severity depends on the amount of scratching involved.

Over many years, there has been disagreement whether a particular food can have an effect on atopic dermatitis. The people who used the word *atopic* or allergic thought that it did. Those who named the condition neurodermatitis felt atopic dermatitis to be a problem connected with the nervous system or stress. Still others believed the condition was an inherited immune system problem.

Med Meaning

Eczema or **atopic dermatitis** is one of the most distressing skin problems. It is estimated that as many as 40 percent of eczema patients have food-related problems. Eczema starts with an itch that causes scratching, followed by a rash. For this reason eczema is referred to as the itch that erupts into a rash. Doctors commonly use the term *atopic* to describe a group of medical problems "without a place," meaning this skin condition is not classifiable into any category in particular, and the factors involved— family histories, stress, and environmental factors, including foods—change with the patient's age.

It turns out everybody is correct—but not merely one thing is responsible. Yes, atopic dermatitis is an inherited condition; but environmental factors, too, can be instrumental in this condition. One factor of our environment is our diet.

Like all food-related allergy problems, there are few accurate, safe tests other than observation and elimination diets (see Chapter 8). The number of times or percentage of times that food is related seems to vary. Some feel that in children with eczema, food plays an important part in 40 percent of the cases. Others say 10 to 20 percent are food-related.

What we do know is that in infants, children, and some adults, food can increase the severity of the condition.

Experts Who Have the Inside Track

Most clinicians feel that food as offender is a more common condition in infants, occurring less as the patient grows older. One theory is that the patient continues to eat small amounts of the offending food, which saturates the immune system's ability to respond with an immediate hypersensitivity (allergic) reaction.

Others disagree, because atopic dermatitis seems to be a cellular immune reaction involving other parts of the immune system.

The elimination and careful reintroduction of food diet technique is the only way to find out whether a food allergy is a factor in eczema. The reintroduction step is sometimes referred to as a challenge. If the food is eliminated from the diet with improvement in the

Skulls and Bones

Eggs, cow's milk, wheat, soy, and peanuts are the foods most likely to cause eczema. Eggs are felt to be the most common cause in that group of foods.

eczema, then the next step is to carefully challenge by adding the food back to the diet. If there is recurrence or worsening of the eczema, then certainly this points in the direction of food as one part of the problem.

Offending Foods

The foods that most often are found to cause problems during childhood are eggs, cow's milk, wheat, fish, soy, and peanuts. Citrus juices such as orange juice may cause more contact problems if the juice gets on the mouth, lips, or cheeks. Shellfish is usually not part of the infant's diet and appears later as a possible problem.

The sources of these foods are discussed in detail in Chapter 6. These are foods that are obvious derivatives of certain food groups.

The difficulty is in learning and looking for those foods where they are least expected. Examples are cow's milk protein in the following:

- Brown sugar flavoring
- Caramel flavoring
- High-protein flour
- Margarine

How about peanuts in chili, chocolate candy, or egg rolls?

Mamma Mia!

A source of food intake in the infant is breast-feeding. Observation has shown that the mother's diet can influence the infant's eczema. This could also be the case in other allergic reactions, such as hives.

Infants have been observed to have an allergic reaction anywhere from 4 to 36 hours after breast-feeding. The mother's diet, including cow's milk, eggs, soy, peanuts, or wheat, can result in a flare-up of the skin condition.

Timely Tip

Nursing mothers must watch their diets carefully, lest their food intake produce food allergies in their infants.

As a result, infants who have a strong history of allergy or who have signs of atopic dermatitis, should avoid cow's milk for the first year of life and eggs for up to two years. Other possible sources, such as peanuts, tree nuts, fish, and shellfish, should be kept out of the diet for two to three years. Naturally, this would apply both to the child and to the nursing mother.

From Scratchy Infants to Itchy Adults

Eczema takes different forms and shapes depending on the patient's age. Infantile eczema usually initially appears between the ages of two to three months up to two years of age. When it does occur, the rash is on the face, cheeks, and chin, especially where the infant drools.

The rash itself is red and occurs in patches. Other areas where it can be found are the front of the arms, the scalp, neck, wrists, and behind the knees. It does not usually appear in the diaper area, because this is a place that is hard to scratch. (Cradle cap or *seborrheic dermatitis* has no itching, and involves the diaper area and scalp).

In the majority of cases, the condition will clear up at around 18 to 36 months of age. Sometimes a viral infection or immunization will increase the symptoms of eczema. The rash itself appears as red areas with raised, blisterlike lesions that are wet or weeping and finely crusty.

The age range for childhood eczema is between 2 and 12 years of age. The skin lesions have less material coming out of the blisters. Now the rash is dry and scaly with raised parts. At this point there can be an even spread of the rash, in which the buttocks and thighs are not spared, as is the case in infancy. An important part of this stage is that there is a thickening or *lichenification* of the epidermal layer of skin.

The areas where the rash commonly appears at this age are places where the person perspires, such as the bend of the arm opposite the elbow, and the area behind the knee. Other areas are the neck, wrist, face, and eyelids. There is also an extra crease below the eyes secondary to constant rubbing called the *Denie-Morgan fold*. The rash of eczema is worse under tight clothing or rough material that can irritate the skin.

During the adolescent and adult stages, the rash is still very itchy, localized in patches, red, scaly, and with raised lesions. The area the rash commonly appears in is still the crease in front of the elbow, neck, forehead, around the eyes, and hands. The problem with the hands is very common, probably because adults wash their hands more frequently. This dries the skin, and the soap plus the rubbing process irritates the skin and makes it even more itchy.

In general, about one third of children with eczema and food-related allergies lose their allergic reaction to the food by three years of age. This is based on a number of factors:

- **The offending food.** Those patients who are allergic to peanuts, tree nuts, fish, or shellfish will not likely see an improvement. Those allergic to soy, wheat, cow's milk, or eggs are more likely to develop a tolerance to these foods.

- **The level of IgE antibodies.** The higher the blood level of IgE to a specific food, the less likely the patient will develop a tolerance to that food.

- **The type of diet.** The degree to which the patient stays on the elimination diet, the better the chance to develop a tolerance to the food.

continues

continued

> Prick-puncture skin tests can remain positive long after the patient develops tolerance to the food. Some physicians will try very carefully to challenge the patient to certain foods at two- to three-year intervals.
>
> A challenge is safer to do with milk, soy, and wheat than with peanuts, tree nuts, fish, or shellfish, as the latter could create a much stronger, dangerous reaction.

Off to a Good Start

Doctors agree that certain foods are more commonly allergenic than others. In children, these foods include cow's milk, eggs, peanuts, wheat, tree nuts, and fish. As the child grows into adolescence and adulthood, the number of allergenic foods increases. Now the list includes citrus, shellfish, and seeds.

In this light, it would seem reasonable to conclude that a nursing mother could reduce the risk of allergies in the newborn by eliminating from her diet those food allergens that have a high allergic potential.

Skulls and Bones

Using drugs, smoking cigarettes, and drinking alcohol during pregnancy do have a bad effect on the developing infant. These actions can cause stillbirth, premature delivery, underdeveloped infants with serious breathing problems, and possibly drug addiction.

The truth of the matter is that strict avoidance by the pregnant mother of foods high on the list of producing food allergies does not totally prevent allergies from occurring in the infant. Studies have shown that pregnant mothers who have strictly adhered to a so-called elimination diet can still give birth to children who later develop allergic reactions to foods. The important factors include the child being exposed to highly allergenic food through diet from the mother's milk, formula, or other environmental exposure. Remember, the creation of a food allergy depends on many different factors.

You Can Make a Difference

Your best bet for decreasing the chances of your child developing a food allergy is in the feeding after birth. As a rule, avoid foods that pose a challenge to the developing infant's still immature immune system and gastrointestinal tract. For example, instead of feeding your baby cow's milk, use a substitute such as hydrolyzed protein formula like Alimentum, Nutramigen, or Pregestimil.

Food Substitutes

Here's a list of food substitutes for foods causing allergies:

- ◆ **Milk.** Enriched rice, soy, or potato milk, calcium-fortified juice, cereal, legumes, nuts, whole grains, dark green vegetables, (source of calcium, Vitamins A and D, protein).
- ◆ **Eggs.** Meat, legumes, whole grains, (source of Vitamin B, selenium, biotin, protein).
- ◆ **Peanuts.** Legumes, meat, whole grains.
- ◆ **Soy.** Not a primary source of any one nutrient.
- ◆ **Wheat.** Enriched and commercial grain from barley, buckwheat, corn, oats, rice, rye, quinoa, and poi.
- ◆ **Fish.** Meat, grain, legumes.
- ◆ **Shellfish.** No substitute.

Patients and nursing mothers who are totally successful with elimination diets must pay attention to their own nutrition. The deficiencies that could occur are calcium, protein, vitamins, and minerals.

The nutrients essential for our diet are in two categories: macronutrients and micronutrients. Macronutrients are proteins, carbohydrates, and fats, all of which are sources of energy. Micronutrients are vitamins, minerals, and trace elements. These can be found in food or vitamin supplements.

Children are more nutritionally vulnerable than adults, because they are growing and need a certain amount of nutrients to accomplish the process. You should watch for any problems by keeping track of your child's height and weight for his age, and measure his/her head circumference. This should be done at least through three years of age.

The best source of nutrition for your infant is breast milk. Breast milk supplies your infant with immunoglobulins that your baby has not started to produce on its own. These immunoglobulins include IgA as well as IgG, which helps fight infection. Because it takes an infant about six months before it is able to fully produce these vital immunoglobulins on its own, doctors recommend mothers breast-feed for at least six months. This will give protection to the infant, especially in a family with a strong, proven history of allergy. Breast-feeding for one year is optimum. By that time, the infant will have developed full adult levels of IgA, IgG, and IgM.

The Importance of IgA

How a food allergy or food sensitization occurs in the infant has to do with the presence or absence of an immunoglobulin called IgA. When an infant is born, it does not have any of its own IgA and none has passed from the mother during the pregnancy. Some IgA is first passed on to the baby in the early stage of breast-feeding. This first breast milk is called *colostrums*. The IgA is needed in the baby's gastrointestinal tract to protect it from invasion by bacteria and other foreign material, such as foods to which it has never been exposed, including cow's milk, egg protein, peanuts, soy protein, grains, or fish. If the IgA is present in the secretions of the stomach, the IgA will attach to these proteins and make them a larger molecule. The larger the molecule, the more difficult it is for the protein to leak through the wall of the baby's gastrointestinal tract into the circulation. If the large food protein particle does get into the circulation, the protein can set up the food allergy.

The infant starts making its own IgA at birth, but does not have enough to really protect itself until it is about six months of age. So to prevent food allergies from the start, it is best to avoid the most common allergy-producing foods until the infant's gastrointestinal tract can protect itself.

Equally important in this attempt to reduce the risk of food allergies in the infant is to pay attention to what the nursing mother eats. Most pediatricians and allergists agree that cow's milk, eggs, peanuts, fish, and wheat head the list of problems. Cow's milk, protein, and ovalbumin from eggs appear in breast milk within two to six hours after the mother eats those foods, and stay in the breast milk for one to four days. During that period of time, food molecules retain their allergy-producing structure. Also, the infant has the ability to produce specific IgE against these foods with the first exposure.

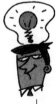

Bet You Didn't Know

If an infant has a respiratory problem called *bronchiolitis*, a family history of allergies, and an elevated IgE in the umbilical cord blood, there is a better than 50 percent chance of allergy problems, including food allergies.

In addition to cow's milk and eggs, nursing mothers should also beware of cereal, peanuts, and shellfish. This results in a very restricted diet for the nursing mother—one that is difficult to follow for one year, and will probably discourage the nursing mother from continuing. However, the benefit to the baby should be worth the inconvenience.

Breast-Feeding A to Z

Health-care specialists are available to teach mothers about breast-feeding. The advice they give is to start preparing for breast-feeding long before the baby is born.

Frequent nursing can irritate the tissue around the mother's nipple, leading to cracking and bleeding. To prevent this, specialists advise taking instruction classes or reading about breast-feeding techniques.

In addition, they advise toughening the skin around the mother's nipple by rubbing it first with soft, and then harder and rougher material. This will help avoid the cracking of the skin that can happen at the start of breast-feeding.

The recommended frequency of breast-feeding is to feed on demand. The baby will let you know when he or she is hungry. The sucking by the infant stimulates the breast gland to produce more milk. Breast-feeding is best started early. The first feeding can be as soon as four hours after birth.

There is also an advantage to having the newborn in the room with the mother so that both are available for each other, to initiate and perpetuate this ongoing relationship.

Skulls and Bones

The oil used to treat the mother's nipple is called *Arachis oil*, which is a peanut product. This same oil is used in a cream to treat cradle cap and diaper rash. These are sometimes suggested by caregivers, and would expose the infant to peanut protein at a very young age.

Timely Tip

Many new mothers who are having difficulty breast-feeding have found help from La Leche League, a national group that is dedicated to promoting breast-feeding. If you need assistance, La Leche League volunteers will even come to your house to help coach you along. For more information, go to www.lalecheleague.org.

The Great Formula Debate

If the infant isn't breast-fed, or if he/she needs supplemental feeding, or it is time to end the breast-feeding, then the next step is a formula that should be something other than cow's milk or a cow's milk-based formula. Alternatives include the following:

- **Soy-based formula.** Some clinicians feel that this is a relatively safe choice, while others feel that there is a high percentage of crossover between cow's milk and soy allergies.

- **Protein hydrolysate formula.** One method of formula-making is to hydrolyze and filter milk-based formula, which will change the protein, making it less hypoallergenic.

Timely Tip

Because the breast-feeding mother is not drinking cow's milk, she should be taking calcium gluconate tablets to supplement her diet, as well as supplemental vitamins and minerals. See the list of food substitutes high in calcium.

◆ **Whey-derived formulas.** A new process will hydrolyze the whey part of the milk. Whey is the liquid part of the milk after it's been curdled. This is found to be an imperfect formula, because it has not totally removed all of the allergenic proteins.

Med Meaning

Hydrolysates are cow's milk treated with digestive enzymes to break down milk protein.

◆ **Casein-derived formulas.** Casein-derived formulas, also known as casein *hydrolysates*, are safer than whey-derived formulas, because they contain fewer allergenic components. Examples of casein-derived formulas are Nutramigin, Pregestimil, and Alimentum.

◆ **Amino acid-based formulas.** Members of this group completely avoid cow's milk as a base, and go straight to using amino acids as the source of protein. Such formulas have been proven safe and effective for infants with cow's milk allergy. Examples of this type are Neocate and EleCare.

As a rule, before choosing a noncow's milk formula for your infant, it is best to consult with your physician. Potentially, an absence of the vital nutrients from dairy products could deprive your child of much needed calcium for growth and bone repair. Calcium is also very important in the functioning of our cells. Leafy green vegetables, vegetables such as broccoli, as well as lentils and peas, are a good source of calcium.

Slow Road to Solids

As your infant grows older, you will have to introduce solid foods. What to give your baby and when are both important factors.

Here are a few pointers to keep in mind when introducing the potentially allergic infant to solid foods:

◆ In the child with a strong family history of allergies, it is best to withhold solid foods for the first four to six months. At that point, solids can be introduced, but only one at a time.

◆ It is best not to give a new food for three days following the preceding solid, to see if there is any allergic reaction to this new food.

◆ If solid foods are started at 6 months of age, the foods given should not be those that are known to be most commonly allergenic.

◆ At one year of age, foods such as cow's milk, wheat, soy, corn, and citrus should be given in small amounts, introduced one at a time in three-day intervals.

◆ The last foods to add to the diet should be eggs, peanuts, and fish.

Some allergists actually advise that peanuts and tree nuts should be avoided until three years of age. This caution is given because of the extreme allergy problems that peanuts and tree nuts can cause. In addition, there is the danger of aspiration of this food into the lungs.

Timely Tip

It is unwise to introduce a new food when a child is ill, because you will not know if any symptoms are from the illness or from the new food.

Stick with the Plan

As we discussed earlier in this chapter, the development of food allergies is multifactorial. Although research has shown that all of the suggestions in this section will help lower an infant's chances of developing food allergies, there is no guarantee that your child will be allergy-free for the rest of his or her life. It is important to repeat that the chance of the baby developing an allergy, including a food allergy, depends on many factors. Many research centers feel these factors include family history of allergy, gender, cigarette smoke exposure, infection, and air contamination with diesel oil exposure.

Allergies can develop at a later age (two to three years). These allergies can include asthma, other respiratory allergies, or eczema. However, some feel that the occurrences of eczema and food allergies are less severe if the food avoidance plan outlined here has been followed for as long as possible.

Suggested Daily Food Intake		
The following table provides an overview of a balanced diet for adults and children on solid foods that is agreed on by certified nutritionists and dieticians.		
Type	**Servings**	**Foods**
Grains	6 to 11 servings	Rice, corn, barley, oatmeal, amaranth, quinoa, buckwheat
Fruits	2 to 4 servings	Fresh, frozen, canned, bottled (source of Vitamin C, potassium folate)
Vegetables	3 to 5 servings	Fresh, frozen, canned, dark green (source of Vitamin A, C, folate, calcium)
Protein	2 to 3 servings	Chicken, beef, pork, turkey, peas, lentils, legumes (source of Vitamin B, folate, calcium, phosphorous, magnesium, zinc)

Baby, You're a Big Kid Now

A strict diet in the nursing mother, plus careful avoidance of highly allergenic food in the child's first one to three years is helpful in reducing the risk of allergy problems early in the baby's life. Nevertheless, even the strictest adherence to suggested guidelines does not completely avoid allergy problems from appearing. What factors can influence the best-laid plans of mice and men?

A child is exposed to multiple factors throughout the growth period, into the adult years. These factors include the family history of allergy; environmental exposure to house dust, mites, and molds; bacterial and viral infections that can affect the immune system; air contamination with pollutants and airborne pollen; cigarette smoke; and medications such as antibiotics and other drugs.

In addition to these factors, caretakers such as baby sitters and nursery school teachers, even grandparents and other family members, can mistakenly expose the allergic child to forbidden foods. Allergens can be on the clothes of caregivers after they have eaten peanuts or tree nuts. Decreased exposure to these factors will diminish the chance of allergic reactions. In real life, however, it's virtually impossible to live within such strict confines; contemporary lifestyles make this impossible.

Bet You Didn't Know

Many authorities feel that the development of allergies is related to environmental exposure. Doctors, for example, agree that exposure to house dust mites and air pollution in infancy do play a part in whether allergies develop in a person later. However, doctors are still debating whether an infant's exposure to pets in the household could influence future allergy problems.

As the child approaches two to three years of age, allergy symptoms can and do occur. They will happen individually or in combination. Eczema usually begins early in infancy, but in some cases it can appear later.

Food allergies typically will have shown some signs by this phase in the child's life. This is also the time that allergic rhinitis, asthma, or gastrointestinal problems might occur.

When Allergy Rears Its Ugly Head

If allergy symptoms begin showing up as the child grows older, the process of diagnosis is nevertheless the same. In the case of food allergies, the method employed is the elimination of suspected food groups (see Chapter 8 for details).

It is very important to observe cause and effect. You should become aware of exposures in the environment that trigger allergic symptoms in your child. Try to answer the questions of what makes allergy worse and what makes it better. A good way of doing this is to keep a food diary to see if any allergy symptoms occur when a certain food is eaten. Eliminate the food, and see if the symptoms disappear.

The next step in the case of a food allergy is elimination and avoidance. This is the same in the case of inhalant allergies. For health care workers, educating the child as well as the parents is extremely important. The more you as a parent know about the problem and its cause, the better you'll be able to handle it and help your child handle it as well.

> **Skulls and Bones**
>
> Be careful not to emphasize or try to convince your child that he or she is different or somehow limited because of his or her allergy. The psychosocial damage is worse than the medical problem. Remember, a food allergy is only one small part of who your child is.

Helping Caregivers Help Allergic Children

Allergies last a lifetime, and can be more severe with each exposure. However, although milk, egg, and wheat allergies in an infant can gradually decrease by three years of age, they may remain on some subtle level. Re-introduction of cow's milk, eggs, and wheat can be tried at two to three years of age, but it should be tried with great caution and in very small amounts.

Education and awareness by patients and their caregivers is crucial. Caregivers must make sure a child understands the importance of not eating any food that will cause the allergic reaction. Caregivers include grandparents, brothers and sisters, aunts and uncles, teachers at school, and babysitters.

To help caregivers in their responsibilities to protect children and other dependent family members, write up an action plan to give to caregivers in your absence. For example, a schoolchild's action plan could be kept at the nursery school, preschool, or elementary school. It should identify the child by name, grade, room number, and teacher's name and list the foods that cause allergic reactions in the child, together with the warning signs and symptoms that could occur. The plan should also spell out in detail emergency treatment procedures, including instructions for the person in charge to call 911, and should include instructions on the use of adrenaline and antihistamines such as Benadryl. Should an emergency arise, the caregiver should be instructed to call both the parent and the physician.

> **Timely Tip**
>
> Nurses in the newborn nursery should be made aware if the infant has a strong family history of allergies. If the nursing staff gives supplemental feedings, they should avoid cow's milk or formulas that contain cow's milk.

> **Timely Tip**
>
> Keep adrenaline in a thermos to avoid temperature change.

In general, an action plan for the allergic child may include some or all of the following points:

♦ Educate all members of the staff regarding allergic reactions and the administration of EpiPen. In the case of schoolchildren, be sure to review the action plan periodically during the school year, as well as at the beginning of each year. Substitute teachers and any other part-time help must be educated. Identify the specific food that causes the allergic reaction.

♦ Educate your child's classmates as to the nature of allergic reactions, so that they can alert the teacher if a problem occurs.

♦ Be sure the staff posts your child's emergency health-care plan in the nurse's office, the main offices, the cafeteria, the classroom, and any other appropriate sites.

♦ Be sure EpiPens are always on hand and easily accessible, for example, in the nurse's office, classroom, and the main office.

♦ Inform teachers to notify parents and the school nurse about all field trips, and to carry the required medication on all excursions.

♦ Instruct the caregiver not to provide the food-allergic child anything to eat or drink that is not approved by a parent.

♦ If a reaction occurs, the nurse or other designated person is to be notified immediately. The child's Emergency Health Care Plan will be implemented.

In cases where food allergy reactions are severe, all of these points are important in preventing serious problems. The better caregivers are prepared, the less serious the outcome. Note also that this plan is most useful for preschool, nursery school, and regular school. It can be adapted for summer camp, trips with other families, or sleepovers at a friend's house.

The Least You Need to Know

♦ There is no one way to identify a newborn who will have allergies.

♦ The best protective measure for a baby born into a family with a history of allergies starts with breast-feeding and also depends on the time solid foods are introduced.

♦ There are good, safe substitutes for cow's milk.

♦ Observation, self-education, and avoidance when possible are the best treatments for allergies.

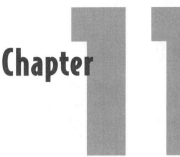

Chapter 11

Dealing with Food Problems as You Grow Older

In This Chapter

◆ Allergies might come or go with age

◆ The problems with allergy medications for the elderly

◆ Advice to caregivers of the elderly

Aging is an unavoidable fact of life that, like it or not, happens in the best of families. Nobody wants to get old, but as much as we may ignore—especially during our youth—the inescapable fact that all of us do age, and no matter that we might believe it will never happen to us, sooner or later, if we live long enough, we, too, will get on in years.

Aging brings a host of new challenges, as we find ourselves increasingly susceptible to more and more health-related problems. For some who've never experienced a food allergy reaction before, it's never too late. Food allergy can strike after 50, 60, 70, and beyond. So let's take a look at how a food allergy may impact you or your elderly family member, and what can be done about the problem.

What, Me Old?

Today, 33 million Americans are over 65, and in another quarter-century, the number will have doubled. Now that our population is living longer, it's not uncommon to see people in their seventies, eighties, and nineties who have more than one medical condition at the same time, so treating older food-allergy patients who have additional issues to contend with is a major concern. If you're a senior with a food allergy, chances are this is not your only medical problem.

The majority of patients aged 50 years or older with food allergies have a history of pre-existing conditions; some, however, begin unexpectedly suffering from food allergies late in life. When an allergy strikes older adults with no previous history of the disorder, a full medical workup will be indicated. This means your physician will order blood and urine tests, plus any follow-up tests that are recommended after preliminary results are in, in order to determine whether your adverse reactions to food constitute a true food allergy.

At later stages of life, many suspicious symptoms require investigation; your reactions could be caused not only by a food allergy but by other disorders that occur more frequently as you age, the symptoms of which resemble a food allergy. Your physician will help you understand if you have a food intolerance or vagus nerve reaction, for example, or if you may have another systemic disorder. Because many concurrent conditions are possible with increasing age, your physician must take all this into consideration, and because more than 70 percent of seniors are on some form of medication, the risk of harmful interaction of food-allergy medication with other medication is greater if you are in this age category.

Your doctor will have to look at the effect of medications you are already taking, and advise appropriate tests any time your pre-existing patterns change.

Timely Tip

If you are the caregiver of an elderly person, make sure your elderly loved one is not overmedicated. Go over all drugs prescribed by his or her physician and/or pharmacist to be sure there are no conflicts or dangerous drug interactions. Some ophthalmic medications (for example, beta blockers) used by older folks have poor drug interactions with specific antihistamines that could be prescribed for food allergy, or with respiratory conditions that may be caused by food allergy, such as asthma or allergic rhinitis, so caution in selection of antihistamine therapy is always necessary.

Lurking Dangers—Age Makes It Worse

As medical conditions such as food allergies strike or worsen with age, treatment must be specially tailored for the older person, due to slower metabolism and the potential for side effects. As you grow older you will have very special needs, so the management of your food allergies, together with any other existing conditions, will ideally be individualized, with medication dosage prescribed accordingly.

Something to watch out for: Drugs typically given to older people often cause drowsiness, affect the balance, and may even accelerate cognitive decline. Many additional pitfalls exist for the senior, far more than for younger people.

Multiple Med Misery

Lacking an effective alternative, many elders consume large amounts of analgesics. An analgesic is any medicine intended to kill pain. Over-the-counter analgesics (medicines bought without a prescription) include aspirin, ibuprofen, naproxen sodium, Tylenol, and others. Often, taking even these common painkillers is dangerous for the stomach, liver, and kidneys; most drugs that can cause kidney damage are the ones that are excreted only through the kidneys. Case reports have attributed incidents of acute kidney failure to the use of such painkillers, including aspirin, ibuprofen, and naproxen.

Your primary care physician as well as allergist and any other specialists you consult will consider existing syndromes to coordinate a total approach to your food-allergy therapy. If you're taking medication for food allergies together with medication for other medical conditions, some of the serious side effects that can result from drug interaction gone wrong include cardiac irregularities, memory loss, lethargy, ambulation instability, blurred or impaired vision, tinnitus, and even fatality.

Topical nasal steroids and antihistamines taken for food allergies provide effective treatment. Since studies show that sedating antihistamines can cause drowsiness and negatively impact thought and function, guidelines for the elderly suggest the use of nonsedating agents such as second-generation medications like Allegra (fexofenadine).

An area of concern for older adults who inhale steroid medicines such as Beclovent, Flovent, Qvar, or other inhaled steroids over a long period of time is that their use may increase the chances of developing glaucoma. Other corticosteroid medication is a concern and should be monitored by your doctor.

Bet You Didn't Know

Food allergies are common problems encountered in the elderly. The conditions of allergic rhinitis, pruritus, urticaria, and anaphylactoid reactions often require H1 antihistamines.

Timely Tip

If you are over 50, it's especially important to have your eyes checked on a regular basis. Glaucoma may result from certain allergy drugs such as oral or inhaled corticosteroids like Prednisone. Glaucoma is irreversible, although it can be arrested. See your ophthalmologist for testing. Patients on long-term corticosteroids should be monitored for cataracts.

Ole Blue Eyes, Ole Brown Eyes

Glaucoma strikes older people in large numbers, and often can be the result of side effects of asthma treatment. Visual symptoms may include blind spots, blurred vision, or decreasing peripheral vision. Nausea and vomiting may also occur.

Glaucoma is caused by the buildup of fluid in the eye due to impaired drainage, which in turn leads to elevated pressure within the eye. This pressure causes pain around the eye, and a glaucoma headache may result. Those at increased risk for glaucoma include people with a history of long-term steroid use and/or a family history of glaucoma in a parent.

Infections and Incontinence

Some medications taken by the elderly may lead to urinary incontinence. Diuretics (used to increase urine output) and drugs with cholinergic effects (as in many antihistamines), have side effects in the urinary tract that may cause bladder spasm and difficulty in urinating. Cholinergic drugs are those that inhibit the secretion of acid in the stomach, production of saliva, and bronchial secretions.

The Elder Itch

Itching is another problem that often worsens with age. Although some itchy skin may be due to hives or eczema, you will want to make sure your problem is not due to nonallergic causes aggravated by the aging process. Whether the cause is a food allergy or other, your doctor may recommend over-the-counter medications such as Benadryl and hydrocortisone to alleviate the itchy condition.

Hives, one of the most common symptoms of food allergy, are red, itchy welts that usually appear on the skin, but also sometimes form in the soft tissue of the mouth, eyes, and throat. The allergic reaction that produces this annoying condition is caused by histamine, released when the immune system tries to fight a foreign substance, which in the case of a food allergy is usually a protein.

Hives may be treated with antihistamines such as Diphenhydramine, Cetirizine, or Loratadine; oral corticosteroids such as prednisone; and epinephrine when anaphylaxis occurs. Both oral antihistamines and oral corticosteroids have side effects such as drowsiness, dry mouth, constipation, and the inability to urinate, and can cause more severe reactions in older people.

If long-term use of antihistamines due to a food allergy is anticipated, physicians will evaluate therapy with the potential for drug and disease interactions, especially in the older patient. For this reason, attention will be directed to use of antihistamines that do not exhibit cardiac or central nervous system side effects.

Higher doses of topical anesthetics than are available without prescription produce relief for only about 45 minutes. Topical antihistamines provide mild relief and are useful for short-term treatment. Decreasing itching can often be accomplished with use of H1 receptor antagonists such as hydroxyzine, loratadine, or fexofenadine (Allegra).

> **Timely Tip**
>
> Allegra is a highly selective H1 receptor antagonist of histamine with few negative side effects such as drowsiness. No doubt you have seen this popular drug advertised in TV commercials.

Every Breath You Take

As you have read in earlier chapters, food allergies cause symptoms affecting the skin, gastrointestinal and respiratory systems. For those whose food allergies cause respiratory problems, such symptoms are especially tough on older people. Reactions may become aggravated in later years, and medications prescribed for their treatment must be monitored very carefully. One allergic respiratory condition of concern which may be aggravated or caused by foods is rhinitis.

Rhinitis is the inflammation of mucosal membranes of the nose. Physiological connective-tissue and circulatory changes in the nose related to aging may predispose an elderly person to rhinitis; then eating a specific food to which one is allergic can aggravate the condition, as can eating very hot food like hot soup or very spicy food like hot peppers.

Allergic rhinitis includes symptoms of pruritus, nasal congestion, sneezing, and runny nose. Antihistamines play an important role in its treatment. Histamine contributes to most of the symptoms, which usually improve with the use of H1 receptor antagonists. These are typically combined with nasally inhaled corticosteroids or cromolyn as anti-inflammatory agents, and if appropriate, topical decongestants may be recommended. However, the latter are not generally used for more than three days at a time, because their overuse may lead to rebound congestion.

The Anguish of Asthma

In the last 20 years, there has been a severe outbreak of asthma in the United States, the reason for which is unknown, although allergies to foods serve to aggravate the condition. Why this has happened remains a puzzle. Asthma is responsible for more than 6,000 deaths per year in the United States, and is the ninth leading cause of hospitalization. More than 17 million Americans suffer from asthma, representing a 75 percent increase since 1980. Of these figures, there has been a substantial increase in asthma cases among older adults. But the normal effects of aging can make asthma in the elderly harder to diagnose and treat.

Asthma diagnosis in patients over 65 is sorely inadequate; 50 percent of elderly asthmatics are undiagnosed, and only 30 percent of diagnosed patients are treated properly. That finding may help explain why the asthma death rate in adults over 65 is ten times the death rate in younger adults.

Blame It on Age

Phrases such as "It's only age" or "You're just getting old" are no consolation when your airways begin constricting and you're gasping for breath. Yet partly because of the misperception that wheezing and difficulty breathing are an inevitable part of aging, asthma remains underdiagnosed in the elderly. Doctors must keep in mind the food-allergic cause of asthma, particularly in the elderly; older persons with asthmatic symptoms caused by food allergies often have higher serum levels of IgE, compared to nonasthmatic persons of the same age, triggering asthma in many over age 65. Thus, when you eat a food to which you are allergic, you are all the more prone to an asthmatic reaction.

Unfortunately, all too many elderly asthmatics who do get diagnosed fail to receive proper therapy. Clinical guidelines recommend daily anti-inflammatory medications such as inhaled corticosteroids (Flovent, Vanceril), plus rescue use of long-acting bronchodilators (Formoterol, Salmeterol). Inhaled corticosteroids rarely cause side effects, and minimize the need for chronic oral corticosteroids such as prednisone, which are associated with a high risk of side effects, particularly for the elderly.

The vast underdiagnosis of asthma in the elderly is probably due to the common misperception that asthma rarely appears for the first time late in life and that episodes of shortness of breath in the elderly are inevitable and are usually due to heart disease. Unfortunately for those older, undiagnosed folks suffering from food allergies, their true condition of a food allergy may be the last problem suspected.

Waiting to Exhale

Tests that are utilized in diagnosing asthma include spirometry, which measures the width of air passageways from the lungs; chest x-ray; electrocardiogram (to rule out heart disease); and blood test.

Treating elderly asthmatics can present complications when treatment interacts with the treatment of other conditions of aging. A method of treating asthma is the use of steroids only when it is necessary. Cortico-steroids can cause serious side affects, such as osteoporosis, stomach bleeding, elevation of blood pressure and blood sugar levels, cata-racts, glaucoma, and skin lesions that heal poorly. Oral steroids are not frequently used to treat food allergies on a long-term basis. The best treatment is avoidance or elimina-tion from the diet.

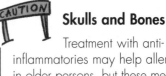

Skulls and Bones

Treatment with anti-inflammatories may help allergies in older persons, but these medica-tions can cause increased kidney and gastrointestinal toxicity.

Calling All Caregivers

A food allergy suddenly appearing later in life can be frightening to you or the older person in your life.

Today, more than seven million households contain caregivers. If you are the caregiver, it will fall on your shoulders to monitor the patient's or your elderly loved one's food intake and oversee everything in his or her diet, to try to work within food allergy parameters.

With the elderly population expanding dramatically, and the over-85 segment growing the fastest, proper nutrition is increasingly important for the health of an aging soci-ety. The use of multiple medications, some of which may be necessary for food allergies, can affect eating patterns in the elderly, as some medications suppress appetite or inter-fere with the absorption of vitamins and nutrients. When diseases interfere with ade-quate nutrition, they cause the body to require more energy, causing the excretion of nutrients by the kidneys. In this case, you will have to make sure adequate nutrition is included in the diet.

Timely Tip

As people age, they are sus-ceptible to loss of faculties and may not be able to make decisions. You must recognize this when it happens to your loved ones, and make decisions regard-ing their health and welfare accordingly.

Long in the Tooth, Short on Memory

With declining faculties, it's possible that your elder relatives will completely forget they have a food allergy, in which case it may be your responsibility to remember for them, and to monitor everything that goes into their mouths. Eating out, travel, and visits to others' homes complicate things even more.

In dealing with their food allergy, it's vital that elderly patients be restrained from eating offending foods. Your loved one may genuinely forget, or on the other hand, might deliberately indulge, just to be defiant and stubborn. A depressed person may even eat offending foods as a self-destructive measure.

Oldies but Not Goodies

Members of the older population are at increasing risk for a stroke. A stroke occurs when a blood vessel to the brain bleeds in a cerebral hemorrhage, or is blocked by a blood clot, which is a thrombotic stroke. If a blood clot travels to the brain from another part of the body such as the lungs and blocks an artery in an embolic stroke, this blockage will interfere with the blood supply to the brain thus causing death of the cells. This is called an infarction wherever it occurs in the body.

Bet You Didn't Know

Dementia, including Alzheimer's disease, is a global problem affecting about 18 million people worldwide, according to the World Health Organization. The number of people with the disorder is expected to increase to 34 million in 25 years' time.

Some of the associated symptoms of a stroke include the exact same symptoms of an allergic reaction to foods—vomiting, dizziness, weakness, and breathing problems. So you as caregiver for your older family member will have to be on the lookout for these symptoms as well, and make sure of the difference.

Home Away from Home

A part of gradual decline in the elderly may be Alzheimer's, dementia, or other neurological conditions. When serious symptoms strike, your loved one may end up needing long-term care. Although only 5 percent of people over the age of 65 live in nursing homes, there is a 20 percent chance that people who live to 65 will spend some time in a nursing home before they die.

Long-term care may be necessary when the elder declines physically or mentally. Most assisted living, rehab, and skilled nursing facilities have an on-site staff who can assist with diets and medications. The health-care team is required to monitor patient status closely, and to look for and address problems of food allergy reactions.

When your elderly family member is admitted to a nursing home or assisted living facility, the staff will ask if he or she has any food allergies. You will also be advised to bring a patient medication list, so that the facility may best serve your loved one.

Laughter Is the Best Medicine

Laughing has been found to lower blood pressure, reduce stress hormones, increase muscle flexion, and boost immune function by raising levels of infection-fighting T cells, disease-fighting proteins called gamma-interferon and B cells, which produce disease-destroying antibodies—which in turn affect the immune system and immuno-globins. Laughter also triggers the release of endorphins, the body's natural painkillers, and produces a general sense of well-being. If you can laugh at life, you'll be that much better able to cope with food allergy problems at any age.

Laughter is infectious. Hospitals around the country have incorporated formal and informal laughter therapy programs into their therapeutic regimens. In countries such as India, laughing clubs—in which participants gather in the early morning for the sole purpose of laughing—are becoming as popular as Rotary Clubs in the United States.

Humor is a universal language. It's a contagious activity and a natural diversion. It brings other people into one's orbit and breaks down barriers. Best of all, it's free and has no known side reactions.

Try to get your loved one to see the brighter side of life, and if you can laugh together—even laugh at food allergy problems—so much the better. And as you help your elder, remember that you are laying a valuable foundation, preparing for your own future.

The Least You Need to Know

- The elderly are susceptible to far more health problems than younger people.
- Age brings inevitable changes; you need to understand these to help your elderly loved one.
- Mental and physical conditions may interfere with allergy care.
- People become increasingly subject to more unsafe drug interactions as they age.
- Because the elderly have very special needs, their management and treatment needs to be individualized.

Chapter 12

Managing Food Problems in Pets

In This Chapter

- ◆ Diagnosing and treating food allergies in pets
- ◆ Learn when pet diets work and when they fail
- ◆ Discover what's really in pet food
- ◆ Find alternatives to supermarket pet foods

The human-animal bond is incredibly strong; our devoted pets are an integral part of the family; they ease their way into our deepest affections to fast become our best friends, giving us unconditional love, companionship, and trust. Naturally, as attached as we are to them, we're concerned for their welfare. When a beloved dog or cat scratches, licks, and chews at himself or herself, you as pet guardian have cause for concern; if your pooch or kitty has frequent diarrhea, ear infections, and vomiting, you suspect something's wrong. Could it be allergy to a food they're eating? For yes, indeed, just like humans, our animal companions can and do develop food allergies and intolerances. It's good to know that your pets' allergies can definitely be controlled, just as human allergies can. This chapter explores how you might control allergies in your domestic animal companions.

Scratch and Tell

Pet allergies are immune reactions in which the animal responds abnormally to what might otherwise be an ordinary substance. Allergic animals, just like humans, possess antibodies that react with specific allergens to produce a series of chemical reactions that cause an allergic response. The underlying biological responses to allergies are the same in your pets as in yourself.

Because animals can't tell you what's irritating them, it's up to you to observe their behavior and discover the source of their problem. Food sensitivities in pets usually first show up as itchy skin. Your cat or dog may shake its head, lick and chew its limbs and paws, gnaw at its tail, rub its face on the carpet, develop scabs and ear irritations, exhibit signs of vomiting, diarrhea, flatulence, or sneezing. It may have runny eyes and nose, rashes, hair loss, develop asthmalike symptoms, lose its appetite, show behavioral changes, become hyperactive, or even have seizures. Because not all of these signs can be attributed exclusively to an allergy, and because you will have to rule out certain problems, it's important at this stage that your pet be diagnosed by a veterinarian.

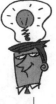

Bet You Didn't Know

The American Veterinary Medical Association says that 70 million cats and 60 million dogs now live in American households. Pet docs estimate the percentage of pets with true food allergies is about the same as for humans.

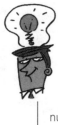

Bet You Didn't Know

No food source is completely nonallergenic. The only hypoallergenic foods are those a pet has never before eaten. To be hypoallergenic, a diet must contain proteins that have been broken down sufficiently so that the immune system does not recognize them. If you have questions about a pet food, contact the manufacturer, whose address is required by law to be on all pet food labels. You may also find a toll-free number as well as a website address listed.

The Cat's Out of the Bag

Veterinarians agree that pets can become allergic to any component of their food; however, the most common offenders are poultry, beef, dairy products, eggs, soy, wheat, and corn. Vets say that proteins in beef, dairy products, and wheat account for two thirds of food allergies in dogs; beef, dairy products, and fish account for almost 90 percent of food allergies in cats. Other allergens implicated include pork, lamb, whey, yeast, preservatives, beef by-products, and tuna. However, any protein-containing foodstuff can be an allergen.

We don't know exactly how many of our four-footed friends have food allergies or food intolerance, mainly because so many owners neglect the problem. However, veterinarians believe adverse food reactions account for 10 to 20 percent of pets' allergic responses, and that food allergies are the third most common allergy in dogs and cats, after inhalant allergies and allergies to flea bites, which rank as number one.

Pets who develop this problem can be any age, from 2 months up to elderly. Many people assume their pet's allergy is the result of a recent diet change; however, the opposite is true: More than 60 percent of animal patients have been eating the offending food for more than 2 years!

Ruling Out

Although pet food allergies usually appear as skin problems and sometimes as gastro-intestinal upset, and because a variety of diseases have similar signs, other causes must be excluded before a diet is blamed. Conditions that mimic a food allergy that need to be eliminated include the following:

- Ringworm, a fungal infection that may cause scaly patches of hair loss or red, raised skin plaques

- Bacterial skin infection

- External parasites such as fleas or sarcoptic mange

- Contact irritants and allergies

Your vet will perform necessary skin tests for inhaled allergens and fleas.

Bet You Didn't Know

Allergies in pets may commonly be diagnosed by skin testing while the pet is sedated and various allergens are injected into the skin. A temporary swelling will occur if the pet is allergic to the allergen. Blood tests are of benefit in diagnosing allergies, but an elimination diet is preferred.

Identify and Eliminate

When your vet has determined that your pet's condition is indeed the result of an allergic reaction to food, your next step is to identify the offending allergen and remove it from your pet's diet. In animals as in humans, food allergies can be diagnosed via skin and blood tests; however, such methods are less reliable in pets than in humans.

Med Meaning

Hypoallergenic pet food has had its proteins chopped into pieces smaller than can be recognized and reacted to by the immune system. You can buy hypoallergenic brands of pet food from your vet. Occasionally, you may also find them in select supermarkets and generally always in pet stores.

The preferred way of diagnosing pet allergy is feeding your animal companion an elimination diet followed by a dietary challenge. Simply changing from one pet food to another is inadvisable because so many pet diets contain similar ingredients; besides, switching randomly from food to food would expose your animal to a number of protein sources, making it harder to find a new one. Instead, you must put your pet on a special elimination diet that consists of a *hypoallergenic* brand of pet food (food that is chopped up into very small pieces, too small to create problems with the pet's digestive system) or find a food that contains ingredients your pet has never eaten before, called a *novel protein*.

Keep a Puss 'n' Pup Food Diary

Start by creating a detailed list of your companion animal's diet; include everything your furry friend has eaten in the preceding month and beyond to the best you can recall. The offender is usually beef, chicken, and so on. In most cases, you don't have to worry about minor ingredients. Next, identify foods that have not been fed previously, to form the basis of the hypoallergenic elimination diet, which may consist of such exotic ingredients as kangaroo, venison, rabbit, duck, ostrich, and alligator (probably unlikely your pet has consumed those). The elimination diet served to your dog and cat should be a protein and a starch—for example, one part lamb mixed with two parts rice or potatoes. Foods can be obtained based on venison and potato, kangaroo and potato, egg and rice, duck and pea (recommended for cats), or duck and potato (recommended for dogs). Rabbit, horsemeat, or fish might also be combined with rice or potatoes. All these formulas are available both as canned and dry formulas. No other foods should be fed during this diagnostic period. Distilled or bottled drinking water is preferable to tap water at this phase, in case your pet is allergic to the water it has been drinking. Last but not least, your pet should be confined indoors as much as possible in order to keep it from eating garbage or some other pet's food, or to keep the pet from foraging for wildlife—particularly cats, who as natural hunters may eat birds, mice, lizards, snakes, bugs, and other crawling life forms.

Timely Tip

When changing your pet's diet, add the new food to the old gradually for a few days to avoid upsetting the pet's digestive system.

If you own both dogs and cats, you'll have to keep the two apart from each other's feeding bowls for the duration of the elimination diet period; make sure Rover stays away from feces if he's prone to eating stool, and keep him far from kitty's litter box, too. Believe it or not, some dogs have a taste for cat stools, and even for cat litter!

During the diet trial no unnecessary medications and no edible chew toys (such as rawhides or bones) should be given, and certainly no table scraps.

Eighty percent of food-allergic pets respond to a trial diet at least partially by six weeks. Some respond much sooner; however, some take longer. Of dogs, golden and Labrador retrievers as well as cocker spaniels usually require ten weeks before showing a response, and some could take longer.

Dog breeds who are genetically predisposed to food allergies include bulldogs, Irish and English setters, shar peis, West Highland white terriers, Scottish terriers, cocker spaniels, Labrador and golden retrievers, miniature schnauzers, Lhasa apsos, shih tzus, akitas, Dalmatians, poodles, German shepherds, boxers, beagles, and basset hounds. Often, these breeds have low thyroid, but fail to respond to thyroid therapy because their hypothroidism is a symptom of poor adrenal function. Additionally, shar peis, terriers, scotties, and akitas often suffer from immune deficiencies that manifest as skin problems.

Success! Now What?

If your pet's allergic symptoms disappear during the trial diet, return to the original food for the next several days. If the symptoms reoccur, you'll know something in the original diet is causing your pet's allergic reaction. The next step is to go back to the trial diet, then add one new ingredient each week. For example, if you've finished a diet of kangaroo and rice and you are ready to start challenging, start the pet on chicken one day, beef the next, and so on, until you find what the pet is allergic to. Once you've found the allergen, you can look for a commercial food that doesn't contain that ingredient.

Some pet owners prefer not risking a return to clinical symptoms; in this case, you could stay with the trial diet if your pet remains symptom-free.

To the Pet "Shot Doc"

Failure to respond within the four- to ten-week period indicates one or more of the following:

- ◆ Dietary sensitivity is not involved.
- ◆ Your pet may be sensitive to the protein in its elimination diet.

- Other factors may be contributing to the clinical disease such as an inhalant allergy.

- Your cat or dog may require a longer diet trial.

In this case, you should consult a veterinary allergy specialist.

What about "allergy shots"? Can they help? Some pets may benefit from desensitization injections; however, small improvements can take eight to ten weeks, and periodic injections may be required for years. Some pet food allergies, however, are responsive to anti-inflammatory drugs such as glucocorticoids. Antihistamines may also be prescribed to help control itching and decrease the amount of glucocorticoids that your pet needs.

Just as with people, there is no magic bullet to "stop being allergic." Immunotherapy treatment is a course of injections that builds up your pet's tolerance to the offending allergens. Cortisone, an anti-inflammatory agent and synthetic version of the corticosteroids naturally released by adrenal glands, may be used to suppress autoimmune functions and manage reactions to allergens. Antihistamines may also be used to treat symptoms.

Skulls and Bones

Many owners overfeed their pets—some 25 percent of dogs and cats that enter a pet clinic are overweight; obesity can shorten a pet's life by contributing to degenerative diseases and other disorders.

Some veterinarians, holistic ones in particular, may consider the herb licorice as an alternative to cortisone. Licorice contains glycyrrhizin, a compound similar to these corticosteroids. This effectively stimulates the adrenal glands and introduces anti-inflammatory, antimicrobial, immune-supporting corticosteroidlike actions on the body. As a result, licorice offers relief from itching and inflammation without completely bypassing the body's own anti-inflammatory functions and without seriously compromising the autoimmune system.

Chow Time

Unfortunately, pet food labels are not only confusing but able to hide many evils, and are often misunderstood or ignored. U.S. pet owners spend some $12 billion a year on cat and dog food, but the average owner buys pet food based on a pretty picture on the package, with no idea what the descriptive terms on the box, can, or bag mean.

Just what are "natural," "adult formula," "gourmet," "premium," and "senior" products? Would it surprise you to hear that a number of terms used have no standard definition or regulatory meaning whatsoever?

Nevertheless, pet foods, which are regulated by the Food and Drug Administration's Center for Veterinary Medicine (CVM), are obliged to carry certain information on their labels, including their Association of American Feed Control Officials (AAFCO) profile.

> **Timely Tip**
>
> Nutrition-wise, there is little difference between canned and dry pet foods. However, canned foods average about 75 percent water and are perishable; dry foods can be stored for longer periods.

What's in a Claim?

The use of the term *natural* on the pet food label is often false and misleading (just as it can be with human food). Claims such as "improves dogs' breath" or "recommended by veterinarians" have no regulatory meaning. A pet food definition of "light" or "lean" depends on the moisture content of the food, and the words *light, lite,* and *low calorie* all have the same meaning. Likewise, the words *lean* and *low fat* are interchangeable. *Less calories* and *reduced calories* mean the product has fewer calories than another (unspecified) product, and *less fat* and *reduced fat* mean the product is less fatty than another (unspecified) one.

> **Skulls and Bones**
>
> Many pet food manufacturers use cheap fillers, grains which are not easily digestible by your pet. These provide minimal nutritional value and are excreted; the manufacturer counts the protein in these grains as part of the total protein of the food, even though dogs and cats can't absorb it.

Pet food can be designated as having a "flavor" as long as the ingredient(s) are sufficient to "impart a distinctive characteristic" to the food. Thus, a "beef flavor" food may contain a minute amount of extract of tissues from cattle, without containing any actual meat at all. The digestibility and availability of nutrients is unlisted on pet food labels.

Tricks of the Trade

While there are hundreds of different pet foods available in this country, most supermarket brands are manufactured by the so-called *majors,* who are subsidiaries of huge multinational companies: Nestle (Alpo, Fancy Feast, Friskies, Mighty Dog); Ralston Purina (Dog Chow, ProPlan, and Purina One); Heinz (9 Lives, Amore, Gravy Train, Kibbles-n-Bits, Nature's Recipe); Colgate-Palmolive (Hill's Science Diet); Procter &

Gamble (Eukanuba, Iams); Mars (Kal Kan, Mealtime, Pedigree, Sheba, Waltham's).

Pet foods, being an extension of the human food and agriculture industries, provide a ready-made market for undesirable, leftover slaughterhouse waste and grains considered unfit for human consumption. In short, what you presume you're buying and what you're actually getting may come as a shock. Here is a list of "hidden ingredients," commonly known as *by-products* that you will find in commercial-brand pet foods:

Bet You Didn't Know

The larger pet food companies use feeding trials to assess the nutritional value of the food. They keep large colonies of dogs and cats for this purpose, or use testing laboratories that have their own animals.

- ◆ **Rendered meat.** Meal is a ground or pulverized composite of animal organs and intestines that have been *rendered*, meaning processed for industrial use. While rendering kills bacteria, it may alter or destroy natural enzymes and proteins found in the raw ingredients. Meat "meal" in commercially manufactured pet food is frequently contaminated with bacteria such as salmonella and Escherichia coli, better known as E. coli. Further problems are a result of contamination with drugs, bacteria, mold, or other toxins. You may even find wood shavings in pet food "meat by-products," which by law must not exceed 35 to 40 percent.

- ◆ **Mill run.** This ingredient consists of residue left after the primary food product has been extracted during the milling process. A "corn mill run," for example, is a pulverized blend of corn husk and cobs, left after a milling process has removed the kernels. Grains "unfit for human consumption," and other waste products are added, including hulls and remains from milling, or items not used by humans because of mold, contaminants, or poor storage practices. These, too, will appear as "by-products," "meat-and-bone meal," or similar names on pet food labels. In other words, your Fido or Fluffy may be eating food containing several types of chemicals that have been added.

Skulls and Bones

Cooking methods used by pet food manufacturers, such as rendering, baking, and extruding (a heat and pressure system used to puff dry foods into nuggets or kibbles), may not destroy hormones used to fatten livestock, or the antibiotic drugs and barbiturates used to euthanize animals.

- ◆ **Rancid fats.** Ever notice a pungent odor when you open a new bag of pet food? What you're smelling is rendered animal fat, restaurant grease, or other rancid oil deemed inedible for humans. Restaurant grease, often stored in drums, may be kept outdoors for weeks, exposed to extreme temperatures until "fat blenders" or rendering companies buy the used grease, mix it together, stabilize it, and sell the blended product to pet food companies, who in turn spray it directly onto extruded kibbles and pellets to make dry pet food edible.

Surely, most consumers don't realize the pet foods they're buying contain by-products that often include decayed meat riddled with disease, or that according to many veterinarians, feeding slaughterhouse wastes to animals increases their risk of serious medical conditions.

Where's the Beef?

Has your pet ever unexpectedly experienced a negative reaction to the same brand pet food you always buy? Perhaps that particular batch of pet food now has different ingredients in it.

The nutritional quality of pet food can vary from batch to batch. According to law, pet food manufacturers are only required to meet the exact formulation of ingredients on their label once every six months. So if they're short of fresh meat one month, they can legally substitute meat by-products or by-product meal for the next six months and not have to change the label ingredients or otherwise inform the buyer.

Timely Tip

A common misconception is that animals are only sensitive to cheap food. If your pet is allergic to an ingredient, price doesn't matter. However, one advantage to more expensive foods on the market is that some do not use fillers that are often the cause of allergic reactions.

Dry Run

Like human foods, pet foods are regulated under the Federal Food, Drug, and Cosmetic Act. Pet food ingredients must be listed on the label in descending order by weight. However, the weight includes the moisture in the ingredient, which makes interpretation tricky. A moist ingredient such as chicken, which may be 70 percent water, may be listed ahead of a dry ingredient, such as soybean meal, which is only 10 percent water—yet the soy actually contributes more solids to the diet. Similar materials listed as separate ingredients may outweigh other ingredients that precede them on the list of ingredients. For example, chicken may be listed as the first ingredient, followed by wheat flour, ground wheat, and wheat middlings. The consumer may believe that chicken is the predominant ingredient, but the three wheat products, when added together, might weigh more than the chicken.

Further, terms required are so vague that two different foods could be made with two different ingredients and have the same term on their labels.

With the long distribution channel for pet food from the factory, to the warehouse, to the wholesaler, to the retailer's storehouse, and finally to the retail outlet, the food you buy your pet could be anywhere from 6 months to 2 years old. Even though your brand might have excellent ingredients listed on the label, their nutritional value could be severely decreased and the oils could be turning rancid by the time you purchase the product. Your best bet is to buy a different grade of pet food, such as premium or hypoallergenic, order from the vet or distributor, or make your own.

Doggone It!

Dogs and cats are carnivorous animals, yet many brands of pet food don't list meat as the first, second, or even third ingredient on the label. Check the labels. Look specifically for the words beef, lamb, chicken, liver, and so on by themselves in the list of ingredients, not as "meal" or "by-product."

Do you have to take all this lying down? No, you don't. For your pet's sake, you can fight back. Let's review how.

Timely Tip

Many veterinarians recommend pets take vitamin Co-Q 10 for allergy relief at the cellular level. Also, digestive enzymes may help improve allergic symptoms by replacing naturally occurring enzymes that are destroyed in manufactured pet foods.

Timely Tip

Ask your vet how much to feed your pet. The feeding guidelines on packages, that is, how much to feed your pet each day, is often much higher than it needs to be. While manufacturers argue that pets vary in size and weight and hence the higher recommended portion, they also want to sell more of their products.

Can It

If you are buying pet foods in a commercial outlet, examine the pet food label closely. Look for:

- **The list of ingredients.** Find a product that lists meat or fish as one of the first ingredients.

- **A reference to guaranteed analysis.** This specifies a product's minimum percentages of crude protein and fat, as well as its maximum percentages of crude fiber and moisture.

- **The life stage/nutritional adequacy statement.** This must disclose whether the product is suitable for: "growth/lactation" or "maintenance," as per the animal's life stages. Every product must meet one of these two profiles. Look for the word "feeding" in the life stage claim. This means the food was proven nutritionally adequate in animal feed tests (tests performed on live animals, not tests done using acid).

- **Feeding guidelines.** How much, how often to feed your pet.

◆ **The manufacturer's name and address.** Hopefully, the manufacturer's telephone number is also listed, so you can call with questions and complaints.

Purr-fectly Clear

Here are a few things you might want to keep in mind when attempting to provide a healthy diet for your pet:

◆ One single pet food can't provide all the nutrition a companion animal needs for its entire lifetime. Still, many people choose one pet food and stick to it, day in and day out. Because cereal grains are the primary ingredients in most commercial pet foods, companion dogs and cats eat a primarily carbohydrate diet, and are being nutritionally short-changed.

◆ Table scraps may be dangerous to your pet; even small amounts of certain foods could be fatal. Cats, in particular, have a much different body chemistry from ours and are susceptible to poisoning from a number of human foods. Also because of their different body chemistry and nutritional requirements, cats should not be fed dog food.

◆ Feeding practices recommended by manufacturers have increased animals' digestive problems.

◆ Feeding only one meal per day can cause irritation of the esophagus by stomach acid. Feeding two smaller meals is better.

◆ Urinary tract disease is directly related to diet in both cats and dogs.

◆ An often-fatal heart disease in cats and some dogs is caused by a deficiency of the amino acid *taurine*. Blindness is another symptom of taurine deficiency.

◆ Inadequate potassium in certain feline diets can cause kidney failure in young cats; potassium is now added in greater amounts to all cat foods.

◆ Hyperthyroidism in cats, often a terminal disease, may be related to excess iodine in commercial pet food diets.

Med Meaning

Cat foods are now supplemented with taurine. Research suggests that taurine may also be helpful for dogs, but as yet few manufacturers are adding it to dog food. **Taurine** is a nonessential sulfur-containing amino acid that functions with glycine and gamma-aminobutyric acid as a neuroinhibitory transmitter. In addition to taurine, cats also need vitamin A, niacin, and essential fatty acids.

◆ A prevalent food problem occurs from milk, resulting in lactose intolerance. Although more common with cats, lactose intolerance can be found in dogs, too.

Timely Tip

If you are giving your kitty home-cooked meals, to ensure the need for taurine is met, cooking juices from the meat component of the diet should be fed, or the diet should be otherwise supplemented.

◆ Pet chews made from rawhide, bone, or other animal parts (such as pig ears) are considered "food," but are not required to give a guaranteed analysis, nutritional adequacy statement, or feeding instructions.

◆ Check with your vet before giving pets supplements, whether alone or in a food product. Supplements you take yourself may be inappropriate for your pet.

The Right Stuff

The number of cats and dogs suffering from nutrition-related disorders, food intolerance, and food allergies is way out of proportion to what the case should be. The bottom line is foods made from by-products, cheap and moldy grains, rotted meat, and rendering are not the best and most nutritious you could find for your animal. What are the alternatives?

◆ **Medical/prescription foods.** You may opt for a category of food known as veterinary medical foods, which can be obtained only through a veterinarian. These foods are designed to treat a particular disease or condition. Several pet food companies research and produce various prescription-type diets: Iams, Purina, Hill's Science Diet, IVD, and Waltham are a few.

◆ **Novel proteins.** The market for "limited antigen" or "novel protein" diets is a multimillion-dollar business. These diets were formulated to address the increasing sensitivities and intolerances to commercial foods that animals have developed.

Timely Tip

Always keep canned pet food refrigerated after opening and do not store it in the can, but in a covered plastic or glass container. If you store dry pet food in a container other than its original bag, be sure to wash the empty container with soap and water before adding food from a new bag. The residual fat that settles on the bottom of the container can become rancid beyond its shelf life; spoiled fat may contaminate fresh food added.

These foods are available both as canned and dry formulas:

- **Hypoallergenic food.** This type of food has had all its proteins chopped into pieces smaller than can be recognized and reacted to by the immune system. Some 80 percent of animal companions with food allergies can be maintained on a commercial hypoallergenic diet. Some hypoallergenic diets include "Nature's Recipe," "Sensible Choice" and "Natural Life," none of which contain chemical preservatives.

- **Hydrolyzed protein diets.** These diets include IVD Limited Diets; Hill's Z/D and Ultra Z/D diets; CNM HA from the prescription diet division of Purina; and Exclude, by DVM Dermatologics.

- **Premium pet foods.** Premium pet food brands tend to use more natural, wholesome, and consistent ingredients in their food. Premium pet foods don't use fillers, so your pet gets more nutrition from an equal serving of a premium brand. This means you feed your pet less food, but more nutrition is retained.

Premium pet foods contain healthy ingredients and do not contain additives or preservatives. Some of the better-known premium pet food companies include: Precise, Eagle Pack, ProPac, Diamond, Life's Abundance, Flint River Ranch, and Nutro, but there are many others. Some of these brands are sold in health food stores and all can be found over the Internet. Recently, some of the leading supermarkets have begun selling their own brand of premium pet foods. Check to see if yours does.

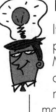

Bet You Didn't Know

It had to happen—you can purchase pet insurance and pet MRIs; pay a visit to pet psychiatrists and pet psychics, and now you can also consult animal allergists, veterinarians who specialize in animal allergy.

Food for Thought

According to the latest research, the ideal pet food consists of protein, carbohydrates, fat, and crude fiber. So the basic nutritional requirements for your pet include …

- **Water.** Of the six vital nutrients, water is the most important. If an animal loses just 15 percent of its total body water, it will die.

- **Carbohydrates.** Essential for energy. Too much consumption, however, can cause obesity.

- **Fats.** An important source of energy, they supply essential fatty acids.

- **Proteins.** For an energy source and for tissue development, such as muscles; and for the luster of the animal's coat.

- **Minerals.** Help maintain fluid balance, cellular operations, and the skeletal structure of the animal's body.

- **Vitamins.** For the maintenance of the body's physiological processes.

Do-It-Yourself Down-Home Cooking

Maybe you're turned off of store-bought pet foods. What can you do? You may prefer to make your own pet food. This is not a difficult or time-consuming process. The four parts to a well-balanced pet diet are: proteins, grains, vegetables, and supplements.

- The protein could include any one of the following: cooked lean beef, chicken, lamb, or fish, which can then be mixed with eggs, cottage cheese, tofu, or cooked soybeans.

- The grain may be cooked rice, cooked potatoes (with the skin), or cooked noodles.

- For veggies, try raw or steamed carrots, cooked broccoli, or string beans. Alfalfa sprouts are good for the skin and can reduce dryness and flaking.

- Supplements may include the following: Olive oil, potassium chloride (salt substitute), and bonemeal tablets or calcium; zinc, silica, and sulfur will help skin problems; fatty acid supplements rich in Omega 3 and 6 help maintain a healthy coat and skin; vitamin C helps provide immunity to disease and may have an antihistamine effect; antioxidant vitamins A, B, and E and selenium are recommended, and seaweed for trace minerals is also helpful.

Homemade pet food eliminates the potentially dangerous ingredients your pets could be consuming from store-bought products.

The Least You Need to Know

- Pets can develop the same food allergies as humans.

- Food allergies in pets can be treated by first recognizing the offending food and then eliminating it from the diet.

- Pet food labels may be daunting at first, but it's worth trying to understand what they say.

- Pets need a well-balanced diet free from harmful ingredients.

- You may find it worthwhile to make your own pet food.

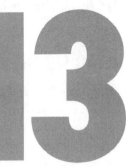

Chapter **13**

Shopping for Allergy-Safe Food

In This Chapter

◆ Learn to decipher food labels

◆ Identify common allergens in unlikely places

◆ Become a smart and alert shopper for allergy-free foods

If you have been diagnosed with a food allergy or intolerance, you must educate yourself on what foods you can safely eat and what to avoid. Alas, separating the tasty from the tasty but forbidden is not always as easy as it sounds—and we're not talking about willpower here (or the lack thereof). Common food allergens such as milk and eggs may be hiding in unexpected fare, and it's up to you to sniff them out, eradicate them from your diet, and replace them with nutritious alternatives. If you want to learn more about common food allergens and the unlikely places where you might find them, this chapter is for you.

Brushing Up on Fruit and Vegetable Bins

An apple a day keeps the doctor away, or so they say. For people suffering from food allergies, however, not every item that shines and beckons from the fruit and vegetable bins of your local grocery store is a safe ingredient of a healthy diet. People with allergies to ragweed, for example, can have allergic reactions to bananas, melons, sunflower seeds, and, would you believe, chamomile tea. Yes, chamomile tea is supposed to be calming and soothing; but it may give you an itchy, tingling mouth. Mugwort, another weed, also can set the stage for reactions to chamomile tea, as well as to celery, carrots, melons, and watermelon.

People with latex allergy commonly also react to bananas, figs, avocados, and other exotic tropical fruits, including passion fruit, papayas, mangos, and pineapples.

Bet You Didn't Know

A protective enzyme called *chitinase* attacks the hard outer skin of insects. This protects bananas, melons, sunflowers, and other fruits and plants against fruit-eating insects. Because this enzyme is common to fruits and plants, it is considered the probable reason or common cause for the allergic reaction.

Timely Tip

Corn is also found in the gum on postage stamps and envelopes, as well as medication in tablet form. Better get some self-sealing envelopes, and don't lick any more stamps.

If you are allergic to almonds, then beware of plums, apricots, peaches, nectarines, and cherries—all of which come with a hard-shelled pit, which makes them members of the same food family.

In spring and summer, strawberries are sweet and tempting. However, be careful how much you eat, because strawberries have a histaminelike substance that in large amounts may cause an itchy welt or two.

Corn has a low frequency of causing food allergy or hypersensitivity. However, there are cases of people with documented reactions to eating corn products. If you have a problem or some uncomfortable symptoms after eating corn, then watch out for corn-based breakfast cereals as well as custard powder, cornmeal, polenta, and sauces that use corn as a thickener. Snacking is a great pastime, but there are those corn tortilla chips. Corn is also hiding behind such names as dextrose, starch (cereal, edible, or food), glucose syrup, hydrolyzed protein, vegetable protein, and many other aliases, so be sure to study food labels carefully. To make matters worse, other cereals containing wheat, rye, barley, oats, rice, or millet can cross-react with corn, causing allergy reactions in corn-allergic people.

Strolling Past the Dairy Case

Cow's milk is advertised in every which way. It truly does taste great with a cookie or chocolate cake. But what about the poor person who is allergic to cow's milk or is lactose intolerant? Even a small amount of cow's milk may cause severe gastrointestinal upset in those unable to indulge in this calcium-rich beverage. The answer is simple: avoid milk, even goat's milk or sheep's milk, at all costs and familiarize yourself with milk substitutes such as water, soy or rice milk, fruit juices, and soy margarine, all of which can be used in baking and cooking recipes that call for milk. If nut allergies are none of your worries, you may also find milk substitutes in creamed coconut, ground almonds with water and honey, and unroasted cashew nuts ground and mixed with honey and vanilla.

If you are concerned that your diet may not be rich enough in calcium, consider calcium-fortified soy milk and gorge on calcium-rich foods such as bok choy, spinach, kale, turnip greens, mustard greens, broccoli, salmon, and sesame seeds (unless, of course, any of these cause you problems).

 Timely Tip

Choose wisely at the deli counter. The staff may be using the same equipment to cut meats and cheese. (And the slicer isn't even kosher.)

Cow's milk is not only found in such obvious dairy products as butter, cream, cream cheese, cottage cheese, curds, custard, ice cream, kefir, margarine, milk powder, sherbet, sour cream, and yogurt, including frozen yogurt; it also hides behind such aliases as whey, casein, caseinates (ammonium, calcium, magnesium, potassium, sodium), hydrolysates (casein, milk protein, whey and whey protein), lactalbumin, lactoglobulin, lactose, and Opta (fat substitute).

If you're looking for butter substitutes, give soy-based margarine, tahini (made with sesame seeds), or sunflower spread a try, provided you are not allergic to these seeds. You might also try clarified ghee, which can be tolerated by most milk-sensitive people, even though it does contain milk protein. People looking for tasty alternatives to cheesy spreads can experiment with soy-based cheeses, tofu, hummus, pate, or taramasalata, a Greek dish of smoked fish roe, olive oil, lemon juice, and garlic.

You also should look for cow's milk in flavorings (such as caramel or coconut cream), baked goods (cake, bread, cookies, crackers, donuts, waffles, pancakes), chocolate, high-protein flour, hot dogs, luncheon/deli meats, pizza, pudding, and pies and pastries with cream filling. Chances are you'll also find traces of cow's milk in commercial bread, cream soup, pancake syrup, fruit snacks, sauces, seasonings, and baby food, as well as canned tuna, which manufacturers enrich with caseinates (a milk derivative) to make it look less like cat food.

In Search of the Incredible, Edible Egg

Soft-boiled, hard-boiled, over medium, over easy, poached, or scrambled—what a great way to start the day. That is, unless you're allergic to these white or brown ovals. Egg proteins and egg white (the most allergenic part of eggs), however, are not only served on a platter; they might also be hidden ingredients in processed meats and other foods. Terms such as albumin, egg solids, egg substitutes, eggnog, globulin, lecithin, livetin, lysozyme, mayonnaise, meringue, ovalbumin, ovamucin, ovomucoid, ovovilen (notice the pattern?), and vitellin all allude to the hidden presence of eggs.

Eggs-in-hiding are brushed on baked goods, found in custard-based recipes, and used in some yogurt and ice cream. You can also find eggs as a clarifying agent in soups and coffee and some wine. Egg albumin (or white) gives shape to fruits that are puréed, and acts as a binder in meatballs and meat loaf. Other scrumptious treats you may have to forgo if you are allergic to eggs include quiche, soufflé, meringue, batter, waffles, Yorkshire pudding, tiramisu, piecrust, mousse, crème caramel, Madeira cake, brioche, marzipan, pastries, éclairs, and most desserts.

A good substitute for eggs is Ener-G Egg Replacer (follow the directions on the box). In your hunt for egg substitutes, you can also find the cooking qualities of egg in gelatin (for puddings, for example). In the case of cookie recipes, you can replace one egg with 2 tablespoons of water, one tablespoon of vegetable oil, and one half teaspoon of baking soda. Additional egg substitutes include:

> 2 TB. corn starch = 1 egg
>
> 2 TB. arrowroot flour = 1 egg
>
> 2 TB. potato starch = 1 egg
>
> 1 heaping TB. soy powder + 2 TB. water = 1 egg
>
> 1 TB. soy milk powder + 1 TB. cornstarch + 2 TB. water = 1 egg
>
> 1 TB. flax seeds + 1 cup water = 1 egg
>
> 1 banana = 1 egg in cakes

Passing on the Nutty Troublemakers

What's better than tree nuts or peanuts at a ballgame or while watching television? Commonly, people who are allergic to tree nuts have an allergy problem with peanuts, even though the two are not in the same food family. Peanuts are a legume just like peas and beans. Peanuts are really a pealike seed that looks like a nut after it's been processed. Tree nuts, like the name implies, grow on trees; peanuts grow under the ground. Tree nuts and peanuts can cause severe allergic reactions, and are usually a lifetime problem.

Reactions to tree nuts and peanuts may be severe enough that a source of injectable adrenalin must be available at all times for those people who are allergic.

Timely Tip

Steer clear of bulk food bins. People tend to spill food from one bin to the next, potentially rendering your favorite treat uneatable.

If you have a nut allergy, remember while shopping that mortadella may contain pistachios, while Mandelonas are really peanuts soaked in an almond flavoring. Oh, and arachis oil is really peanut oil. (*Arachis hyhypoaea* is the Latin name for this legume.)

You should also be suspicious of any product or ingredient with the name "nut" attached, including *NuNuts* (reconstituted nuts). Nuts also lurk in such tasty treats as marzipan and nougat. Sneaky names also include hydrolyzed plant products or vegetable protein. If nuts drive you nuts, also look carefully at the list of ingredients in cereals, crackers, and baked goods.

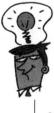

Bet You Didn't Know

Sesame seed, poppy-seed, and cottonseed are found in trail mix, crackers, and buns, not to mention shampoos, conditioners, facial lotions, and styling gels. All those herbal, natural contents of shampoos are sometimes actually a derivative of or byproduct of seeds and weeds. A person allergic to these allergens can have itching, redness, or welts after using these products. Note also that sunflower seeds on many occasions are produced on equipment used for peanut products.

Wise Up to the Seedy, Wheaty Foods

Sesame seeds have become an increasingly popular food source for snacking, as well as a regular ingredient in restaurant fare and prepared meals. You can find these seeds in Halvah (a Middle-Eastern sweet treat), tahini, and sesame oil, as well as on buns, bagels, bread sticks, bread, rice cakes, and veggie burgers. Occasionally sesame is hidden in hummus, stir-fried foods, mixed spices, chutney, salad dressing, cosmetics, and drug preparations. Sesame also is hidden in imported foods behind names such as benne, till, simsim, and anjoli or cengili. Consult your imported food market or cookbook for more information on these products.

Wheat is commonly referred to as the "staff of life"—a label with which those allergic to this grain will have to disagree respectfully as they keep their eyes peeled for this potential troublemaker. Wheat is everywhere; you can find it in breads, buns, and other baked goods and breaded foods, including muffins, nam, pita, pizza, and scones.

You can also find it in breakfast foods, bulghur, couscous, cracker meal, durum, farina, graham flour, gravy thickened with flour, kamut, semolina, soups and sauces, and meat products. Under wraps of secrecy, however, wheat also goes by the names of gluten, glutenized starch, modified starch, cornstarch, enriched or high-protein flour, or vegetable gum. Any "starch" deserves your suspicion.

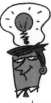

Bet You Didn't Know

The label "hypoallergenic" means anything the manufacturer wants it to mean. There is no standard definition or criteria.

Skulls and Bones

Bleu cheese can contain gluten from the bread used to inoculate the cheese with blue mold.

The gluten portion of wheat is a special problem for those with celiac disease or dermatitis herpetiformis. Gluten-sensitive people should also be very wary of rye and barley in foods or in beer or malt. Additives can contain wheat or barley. Traces of gluten are also found in caramel and caramel color, citric acid, dextrin, gum base, malt flavoring, maltodextrin, and MSG.

If you're still looking at gluten as a problem, then remember that barley enzymes are used in the production of rice milk, some soy milk, soy sauce, and miso. Don't forget that multiple foods such as ice cream, candy, soup, sauce, dressings, cream cheese, and cottage cheese use wheat or other grains as stabilizers.

If wheat is not the "staff of life" for you, you can substitute ⅞ cup rice flour or ⅝ cup potato starch flour in recipes calling for one cup of wheat. You can also try other grains such as quinoa, amaranth, and millet, or arrowroot, rice flour, potato flour, barley flour, rye flour, and sago flour to thicken soups, sauces, and stews. If you prefer to buy rather than bake, look for gluten-free bread, gluten-free flour, rye bread, rye crackers, oat cakes, rice cakes, and rice crackers.

Each wheat alternative adds a slightly different flavor and texture to foods. Selecting a flour is partly a matter of personal choice, and partly what recipe you're using the wheat substitute flour for, whether you're baking breads, cakes, or pies, or thickening a recipe. You should also keep in mind that most nonwheat flours do not substitute cup for cup for wheat flour. Usually, it's a good idea to combine different flours for maximum effectiveness. You might want to experiment in order to find your own ideal combinations.

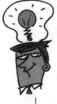

Bet You Didn't Know

The sandwich was invented in England in 1765 by the Earl of Sandwich, head of the British navy (who presumably did not have a wheat allergy).

Look Out for Legumes

Soy products, it seems, are found in almost every prepared food in the grocery. Soy is a good source of protein in our diet-conscious society, and seems to be found on many labels in prepared foods. Pick up any product from soups to nutrition bars, and you will see hydrolyzed soy protein, soy concentrate, soy isolate, and so on. Soy also appears as vegetable gum, vegetable starch, natural flavoring, or lecithin, and soybeans have become a major part of processed food in the United States.

If you enjoy Chinese food, then there's soy sauce and soybean curd. In Japanese cooking, you have miso and shoyu sauce. And of course, there's the ever-present tofu that's used in many high-protein meatless dishes.

Men with prostate cancer are encouraged to include large amounts of soy in their diet, because soy acts like a natural estrogen. However, women being treated for certain types of breast cancer are discouraged by their oncologist (a cancer specialist) from eating large amounts of soy products.

You should also know that soy formula can cross-react with cow's milk allergy in infants. Once an allergy to soy is proven, you must be careful with other members of the legume family, including beans in all shapes and colors—kidney, navy, white, lima, baked, butter, mung, pinto and garbanzo beans (also known as chickpeas)—as well as lentils.

On the Lookout for Something Fishy

There are no helpful hints on fish, other than people allergic to one type of fish can be allergic to others.

Shellfish are categorized in two groups: mollusks—such as clams, abalone, octopus, mussels, oysters, squid, and snails—and crustaceans, which include shrimp, crab, lobster, calamari, prawns, and crayfish. The good news is, patients can be allergic to one group and not the other. The bad news is allergy to shellfish is usually a lifetime allergy—and it often causes a rather severe reaction.

Be very cautious of products that use oyster sauce or clam juice to flavor soups, vegetable purée, or other dishes. Black noodles served in some dishes are really noodles blackened with ink from an octopus. Caponata, a sweet and sour Sicilian relish, might contain anchovies, as does Worcester sauce. Surimi, or imitation crabmeat, contains fish.

Beware of the Sneaky Petes

Even if you are very careful and try very hard to avoid the offending foods, you still are faced with a major challenge of our times—for the most part we no longer make all our foods at home from pure, unaltered raw materials, and the prepared and processed foods we buy are not pure, and the labels are often incomplete due to uncooperative manufacturers. For example, sometimes in the preparation of a food, rolling it in wheat flour is part of the process, yet you will not find wheat listed in the labeled contents. Likewise, natural flavor or artificial flavors can really be milk, wheat, corn, or potato, and added spice sometimes means garlic oil.

Furthermore, you should be wary of seemingly innocent labels such as "may contain," which typically is a dead giveaway that a food has been processed with equipment used to process other foods such as peanuts, and "nondairy," which, due to an FDA loophole, may be applied to foods that contain the milk derivatives casein or caseinates.

Timely Tip

Any time your favorite brands are labeled "new" or "improved" or the packaging changes, reread the label—the ingredients may have changed. For example, one manufacturer of chocolate chip cookies has an egg and nut-free version and another version that contains egg and nuts. Many people would assume that because they can eat the regular brand, they could also eat the chewy or flavored one. Not so.

Kosher symbols on food can help people allergic to dairy products: The letters "K" or "U" found near the product name indicate the presence of milk protein; an "E" on the label indicates the food was made on equipment shared with dairy products. If the product contains neither meat nor dairy products, it is labeled "Pareve," "Parev," or "Parve." Pareve-labeled products indicate that the products are considered milk-free according to religious specifications. Be aware that under Jewish law, a product may be considered "Pareve" even if it contains a very small amount of milk. In other words, it may have enough milk protein to cause a reaction in a milk-allergic person. To be safe, look for "dairy-free" or "suitable for vegans."

As a rule, the FDA requires manufacturers to list ingredients in rank order on the food label. However, when it comes to small quantities—2 percent or less—manufacturers are not legally required to list the ingredients. Instead, these ingredients may be lumped together as "spices" or "flavorings" which may contain almost any food that can trigger allergic reactions in sensitized people. In the food industry, this exception is known as the "2 percent rule."

In general, people who are allergic can't go wrong when they stick to the following rule of thumb: Read the label. If you can't identify the food, if you don't know the total cooking process or all of the ingredients, don't buy or eat the product.

A word about food additives is necessary to round out a discussion of the hidden things we eat yet do not pay attention to. It is estimated that each one of us takes in over 3,000 different additives. These include preservatives, coloring, taste enhancers, and anti-oxidants. The body seems to be able to break down these chemicals without causing any medical problems. From time to time there are warnings about MSG in

Chinese food and food dyes in colored foods. For the most part when these have been looked at critically with blinded and doubled blinded food challenges, the problems or symptoms have not proven them to be reproducible. Metabisulfites, a commonly used preservative in a wide range of foods such as wine, dried fruits, and other foods, can cause severe reactions mainly in people with asthma.

Preservatives include sulfites, metabisulfites, and sulfur dioxide, as well as nitrates and nitrites used in smoked meats. Antioxidants prevent spoiling of fats and oils and are sometimes listed as BHA or BHT. Flavor enhancers include many natural materials such as soy sauce, clam juice, oyster sauce, and ally alcohols used in sweet snacks and soft drinks. Metabisulfite is also a flavor enhancer. Coloring was thought to a problem in the past but recently has not proven to be the ogre we once thought it to be.

The problem with diagnosis is that we have no specific test to help point to one chemical or another. Nor do we know exactly which combinations of these chemicals can cause problems.

Parting Thoughts

Providing a complete list of foods or food products that might be a source of an allergy is beyond the scope of this book. We can list the most common sources and try to make you aware of what to look for in pure and prepared foods. Remember an individual food is only allergenic to the person who has allergies to that particular food. The most common foods that cause allergies are cow's milk, eggs, fish, peanuts, tree nuts, shellfish, wheat, and corn.

If you are suffering from food allergies or intolerance, consult the Food Allergy Anaphylaxis Network (FAAN) at www.foodallergy.org for additional suggestions and monthly updates on this very intricate problem. FAAN also publishes cookbooks and cards for each food group with information on what to look for while shopping. These cards are small enough to carry with you while shopping.

The Least You Need to Know

- Always read food labels in search of hidden ingredients that may cause you illness or discomfort.
- Some people allergic to certain items (such as latex) may also react to similar botanical classes or proteins in certain foods.
- Some allergenic foods are not listed on labels, because of uncooperative manufacturers.
- The Food Allergy Anaphylaxis Network (FAAN) provides handy information to take with you to the supermarket.

Chapter 14

Eating Out—at Home and Abroad

In This Chapter

- How to enjoy an allergy-free meal in restaurants
- What you need to know before you travel
- Airplane, train, cruise and car travel safety rules
- How to prepare for travels abroad

Three-course meals in five-star restaurants, gourmet cuisine in glamorous foreign capitals, buffet fare aboard luxury Caribbean cruise ships, a luau under the stars in Hawaii—don't think you have to forego these alluring pleasures just because you happen to have a food allergy or food intolerance. If you have a mild to moderate food allergy, don't hesitate to go on adventurous backpacking and river rafting trips, sail the Mediterranean, fly to distant, intriguing locations, or enjoy a nice meal at your friendly neighborhood eatery. Admittedly, if your allergy is a serious one, some further strategic planning will be necessary to make things go smoothly. It may be challenging to arrange, but safe dining and travel are possible for the allergy sufferer. This chapter explores what you need to know to enjoy a trouble-free dining experience at home, abroad, or on the road.

To Eat or Not to Eat

Make no mistake—for people with food allergies eating out bears greater risks than eating at home. The numbers speak for themselves: 75 percent of deaths from food allergies involve meals prepared in restaurants and cafes, fast-food joints, food courts, and other commercial outlets, or by outdoor vendors. Estimates are that at least 150 to 200 people a year in the United States die from extreme reactions to allergens such as peanuts, shellfish, and eggs, and thousands more are hospitalized as a result of something they ordered eating out. In fact, to cite Joanne Schlosser, president of the Food Allergy Awareness Institute, 80 percent of deaths due to food allergy result from peanut and tree nut, followed by shellfish and fish.

Clearly, restaurant dining poses a risk, but those consumers who bear the greatest risks are those who are unaware their symptoms could become life threatening. Be that as it may, those who know they are allergic, who do exercise caution but who unfortunately happen to be served cross-contaminated food, do indeed face problems. Believe it or not, in a recent study, over 95 percent of those who died knew they were allergic to the food they consumed. Either they were told the food didn't contain the offending item, or they assumed it didn't and never asked. An added problem in this category are teenagers who know they are allergic but want to be "cool" with their friends, so order something they think is safe but won't ask the server to check, because it wouldn't be cool to ask; or they don't carry their EpiPen and it takes too long to get them emergency treatment.

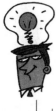

Bet You Didn't Know

People with a nut allergy have died after eating a chicken sandwich, a slice of lemon meringue pie, Italian ice, or a Florence torte, simply because they didn't know the food contained nuts.

Here are a few tips that may help make restaurant dining safer and stress-free:

◆ **Don't eat out on weekends.** Avoid Friday, Saturday, and Sunday, the three most popular days for dining out. Instead, try Monday, the least popular day of the week for eating in restaurants, when the staff can give you more attention. Or dine early before the restaurant is swamped.

◆ **Stick to the tried and true.** When choosing a restaurant in your hometown, it's safer to stick to the proven, tried and true. If you go to a new local spot, contact the restaurant ahead to ensure they have something safe and discuss your needs with a manager before you arrive. When you arrive, introduce yourself to the manager, advise him or her again of your problem, and develop a relationship so that your requests are known. Last but not least, tip generously so the staff get to know and appreciate you. And of course, be sure to thank them for taking such good care of you.

- **Educate yourself about restaurant fare.** Before frequenting a new restaurant, review the menu to be sure they feature something you can eat, and don't be afraid to ask about the ingredients in certain foods. Common food allergens are key ingredients in savory dishes and condiments: A hollandaise sauce is mostly made of butter and eggs (and a twist of lemon); soufflés are prepared with eggs; caponata, a traditional sweet-and-sour Sicilian relish, may contain anchovies, as can Caesar salad dressings or Worcestershire sauce; surimi (imitation crabmeat) is reconstituted, minced fish meat; bisque not only means shellfish but also cream. Note also that after grilling a steak, many chefs use butter to add flavor— the butter melts and becomes invisible and hazardous to those suffering from milk allergy. Chowders may contain fish or shellfish, dairy, wheat as a thickener, and sometimes egg. In some Chinese restaurants, the meats are often dipped in eggwash to make them shiny.

- **Be on the lookout for cross-contamination.** Always ask about how the foods are prepared before you place your order—foods that are safe for you to eat may have been prepared using equipment and tools contaminated by an allergenic food. For example, if you are allergic to shellfish, always ask if the same cooking oil is used for regular fish and shellfish, or if the chef uses oyster sauce or clam sauce or juice to flavor the soup. When ordering onion rings or French fries, find out if the same deep-frying fat is used to deep-fry shrimp. When frequenting restaurants that serve grilled foods, ask if shellfish is prepared on the same grill as chicken and steak. Explain your situation and how they must use clean utensils, grill, etc., to meet your needs. If that is not possible, ask what options they have to guarantee you a safe meal.

- **Inquire about your chain food.** When eating in a national chain, don't be afraid to ask questions before you place your order. Although food preparation is usually standardized, there may be regional differences.

- **Keep it simple.** Order simple meals such as steamed vegetables, baked potatoes, or broiled meat, and steer clear of buffets (people sometimes use the same spoon to serve themselves different foods) as well as covered dishes—you won't know what's in a pot pie until you sink your teeth into it.

- **Think twice about certain ethnic dishes.** If you're allergic to peanuts or tree nuts, avoid Chinese, Thai, Vietnamese, Indian, and African foods; these allergens are a common ingredient in their ethnic dishes. These dishes may also contain many more ingredients than is stated on the menus—mostly for flavorings.

- **Think thrice about seafood restaurants.** If you have a fish allergy, seafood restaurants should be off limits, even if you order a nonfish meal, because kitchen areas may be contaminated by small amounts of fish protein.

♦ **Be sure you're in good company.** Make sure your friends and family know about and understand the ramifications of your food allergy, so they can be of assistance should an emergency arise. If you're single and on a "blind date," make sure your new companion knows about your food problem in advance, and is advised what to do should something unforeseen happen. This may not sound like a great way to start off a budding romance, but hey … at least you may get some good insight into the degree of caring and sympathy of your potential new love. And always carry the appropriate medications, and don't be afraid to use them when needed.

♦ **Don't be afraid to ask.** Servers are not always educated about the foods the restaurant serves; ask to see the manager or maitre d' to be sure, and be specific with the questions you ask. To be absolutely on the safe side, you may want to carry a card that lists the items you have to avoid, including their sneaky incarnations, and show it to the management.

Don't underestimate the risks of eating out. Food products containing allergens can be all but impossible to control in a food service environment, especially if the same equipment and tools are used in the preparation of different foods. However, education and awareness will save the food-allergic person many times over.

Mixed Nuts

Restaurants can be hazardous for those with nut allergies. Even if you explain yourself to the staff, there's always the possibility of cross-contamination—a utensil moved from one pot to another can result in traces of nut transferred to the food you eat. For example, nuts could be transferred from muesli to your plate at breakfast.

Nuts may also show up in foods that appear safe at first. "Artificial nuts" might be deflavored peanuts, reflavored with a nut such as pecan or walnut. Peanuts may be used in some foods with a different name, especially in restaurants that list their menu in another language. For instance, mandelonas are peanuts soaked in almond flavoring.

If you're allergic to nuts, you'll have to avoid salad dressing made with walnut oil or foods cooked in peanut oil; turkey stuffed with chestnut dressing (especially if you're allergic to latex); kaiser rolls, which contain poppy seeds; breakfast cereals containing sunflower seeds; foods containing pine nuts (pignole), such as some pesto in Italian cooking, and so on. You'll also have to avoid hamburger buns with sesame seeds; tahini, and hummus; to complicate matters even further, sesame seed is particularly difficult to avoid with certainty, as the seeds are so small they may easily fall off bakery products onto another food item. A hot curry or jalapeno pepper seasoning can mask the tingling you may get in your mouth if you accidentally eat any food you're allergic to. If you have asthma as well as a nut allergy, you need to take extra care. Asthma is known to increase the risk of death in people with a nut allergy.

Plane Nuts

Peanut allergy is one of the most widely talked about food allergies, and is becoming more and more common. It's also the food allergy most likely to be fatal. Even the smell of peanuts can cause a reaction in a highly allergic person. For this reason, peanut-allergic people often hesitate to fly, particularly in planes where peanuts are served as snacks.

Passengers have had severe reactions to peanuts while flying even when they've not eaten the offending food. Travelers within three rows of the allergic person have offered to abstain from eating nuts, and still the allergic person had a reaction. So how can a nut-allergic person protect him- or herself in the air? Follow these tips:

♦ Let the airline know of your allergy when you book your flight. Arrange to have a nonallergic meal served. Special foods are usually available from some airlines by advance request. If not, bring your own fare to nosh on.

♦ Ask the airline to serve a nonpeanut snack to everyone on your flight. Ask for a written confirmation. Get the names of the people you speak to. Take extra care when using a travel agent to book flights. If the airline does not honor your request, make other flight plans—if the airline is still in business.

♦ Make plans to fly at off-peak times when you're more likely to get better attention for your special needs.

♦ Just to be on the safe side, wipe down seats, armrests, tray, and window area upon boarding the plane. Inspect the floor and remove any food residue from previous flights if a flight attendant is unavailable. If needed, don't be afraid to wear a surgical mask and gloves.

♦ Keep in mind that airlines can't control what other passengers may bring on board—they may carry peanuts on the plane with them. If a reaction occurs, notify the flight crew immediately, so they can identify health professionals on the flight to help you. Every flight is equipped with a medical kit that contains epinephrine.

Timely Tip

The U.S. Department of Transportation has told the airlines they must set aside a peanut-free zone, when requested to do so by passengers with medically documented peanut allergies. The minimum for the peanut-free zone is the row where the passenger sits, plus the rows immediately in front and behind.

Fly Safely

Air travel is generally one of the safest transportation modes. Millions of passengers around the world each year choose this method of travel, the vast majority of whom experience no ill effects from their journey. Nevertheless, planning can often make any trip more comfortable, both during and after the flight. To head off problems before arriving at the airport …

- Pack medicine in a carry-on bag rather than in baggage you plan to check, in case your luggage is lost, stolen, or delayed. Medications should be kept in their original containers.

- Bring along a doctor's note certifying your need for prescription drugs, to avoid being detained by security or customs officers, especially if carrying an EpiPen.

- Carry a summary of your medical records, in case they're needed while you're away.

- Avoid drinking excessive amounts of alcohol the night before flying or aboard the plane. Alcohol dehydrates the body, and the effects are worse at high altitudes. Alcohol will dilate the blood vessels in the area and release histamine as a chemical reaction on the mast white blood cells, aggravating other allergens.

- Ask that sauces and salad dressings be put in individual containers or not served at all. Be sure the airline is aware of your food allergy. Be sure to have a back-up plan like packing safe snacks, in case your request is lost or forgotten.

- Eat before the flight and/or carry your own food onto the plane to be safe. Airplane meals aren't labeled, so you can't know their ingredients. Plan for delay contingencies. Energy bars, fruit, crackers, or other easy-to-carry snack foods come in handy.

Traveling by air can cause or worsen certain medical conditions. Flying takes a toll on the body; there are problems related to changes in air pressure, reduced amounts of oxygen, turbulence, disruptions of the body's internal 24-hour (circadian) clock, and other physical stresses.

Timely Tip

If you're prone to asthma attacks, make sure you have your peak flow meter, nebulizer, or other devices with you when you board a plane. If you need oxygen, the airline can provide it if you arrange it in advance.

Jet planes maintain air pressure inside the cabin at low levels at which air trapped in pockets within the body, such as in the lungs, inner ear, sinuses, and intestinal tract, expands by about 25 percent. This expansion sometimes aggravates medical problems such as respiratory conditions, blocked *eustachian* tubes, and chronic gas pains.

Allergies may produce fluid and swelling that block the eustachian tube, and repeated infections may result in scarring that partially blocks it. Then air becomes trapped in the middle ear, producing pressure (barotitis media) and pain. If you become susceptible to barotitis media, you should chew gum, suck hard candy, or drink something during ascent and descent to encourage swallowing.

Similarly, air may be trapped in the sinuses (barosinusitis), causing facial pain. Swallowing or yawning during the plane's descent and taking decongestants can prevent or relieve these conditions. Take Afrin nasal spray one hour before boarding the plane for take-off and before landing as well. (As Afrin is a 12-hour spray, you may have to adjust these hours to suit your travel schedule.)

Med Meaning

The **eustachian** tube is the passage that connects the middle ear with the back of the nose. This tube is instrumental in equalizing the sensation of pressure in the ears you get at higher altitudes by allowing air to flow in and out of the middle ear.

Alternate Routes

Okay, maybe you're not flying. There are other means of getting from here to there, all of which have their particular pleasures and perils, all the more so if your problem is food allergy. This section examines other modes of travel.

SUVs in Motion–on the Road

Family vacations often involve packing the kids in the car and just taking off. Whether Disneyland or Disneyworld a thousand miles away is your destination, or if you're just planning a simple outing so your parents can visit with their grandchildren, if you (or anyone in your family) has an allergy, extra measures must be taken.

- Know what emergency facilities are available in the area you'll be visiting.

- Call ahead to check out the eating facilities available en route as well as at your destination. Plan for mealtime stops.

- Don't store your EpiPen in the glove compartment—it's heat sensitive. Carry extra emergency kits, and make sure everyone knows where they are and how to use them.

- Plan to start your trip after a meal. Or make it a fun family event by stopping for picnic meals along the road at scenic rest areas, to break up the journey and enjoy safe food.

- If you're staying in a hotel or motel, book a room with a kitchenette and refrigerator so you can cook. Be sure to scour the utensils before using them.

- Avoid staying with people who don't respect your diet restrictions, even if they're family. You can visit with these people at nonmeal times.

All Aboard Amtrak or Go Greyhound

Some families would rather not drive; they prefer trekking via Greyhound or boarding Amtrak to enjoy a hassle-free trip, watching the scenery go by. If you like train rides and opt for Amtrak, you have a choice of taking your meals in the dining car, purchasing a limited choice of packaged meals (mostly sandwiches) from vendors aboard the train, or bringing your own fare from home. (Guess which is safest!)

As far as Greyhound goes, their buses make numerous stops along the way at terminals where available food is mostly packaged goods that are extremely limited in variety. Again, bringing your own food is the best solution for allergy sufferers.

Timely Tip

You may need antidiarrheals when you travel. Medications such as Lomotil or Immodium can decrease the number of diarrheal stools, but may cause complication for persons with serious infections. If you experience traveler's diarrhea, rehydrate quickly by drinking water and other non-sweetened fluids such as soup.

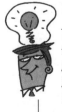

Bet You Didn't Know

The Disney Cruise ships trained their staff using the Food Allergy Awareness Institute's *Serving the Allergic Guest: Increasing Profit, Loyalty and Safety* videotapes.

Ports of Call

Each year, 6.8 million passengers board cruise ships in North America. According to Cruise Lines International Association (CLIA), a nonprofit organization representing 24 cruise lines, the number of North American cruise passengers has increased by 17 percent in the past two years.

Even those ships that don't cater to people on special diets can usually accommodate allergic requests. Because most cruise line food is prepared to order, it's not a problem to get a menu item altered to suit individual needs. Always advise the cruise line ahead of time, especially in the case of severe allergy. One caveat: Cruise ships frequently serve meals buffet style. Don't go there.

The Royal Caribbean Cruise line says they can modify many of the meals on their menu to suit a person with food allergies. Carnival Cruise line would like special dietary requests to be made at least two weeks prior to departure, and also recommends that travelers talk to their waiter about special instructions for preparing menu items. On the Cunard line, any special request will be met, provided the line is notified thirty days prior to departure.

If you have severe asthma, you should let cruise operators know beforehand. Most cruise lines have medical facilities aboard ship; however, it is your responsibility to find out exactly which medical services are available.

V Is for "Virus"

A Center for Disease Control report showed that stomach virus outbreaks on cruise ships tripled the previous year's number and exceeded the last four years combined. Symptoms of the bug, known as Norwalk or norovirus, include nausea, vomiting, diarrhea, abdominal cramps, fever, and headache.

Gastrointestinal symptoms often stem from water and food contamination among groups of people in close contact. It's not hard for viruses to be transmitted from person to person in an enclosed environment like a cruise ship. The fecal/oral virus, which passes from hand to mouth, spreads quickly as passengers touch the same handrails and elevator buttons and use the same public restrooms. Passengers are advised to wash their hands frequently.

The Other Side of the Pond

Of the millions of people who travel out of the country every year, one out of thirty needs medical attention. In preparing for your trip abroad, consulting with a travel medicine specialist has advantages. Doctors specializing in travel medicine obtain bulletins from the World Health Organization, the Centers for Disease Control, and other sources, and have up-to-date, accurate information concerning health conditions around the globe. You'll be advised according to your particular itinerary and medical problems.

Travel is often challenging to the human body. Knowing what these challenges are before you set out enables you to prepare for them. Let's look at some of the most common and easily treatable medical problems you might encounter.

When traveling abroad, translate your allergy situation and needs in writing. (We try to help you do this in our generic letters, later in this chapter.) Carry several copies; give them to the staff to take to the chef. This will help you stay safe. Learn the key words for your allergy when traveling; for example, in

Timely Tip

Iodine tablets and water filters can be used to purify water if bottled water is unavailable at your destination.

Spanish, egg is *huevo*; in French, the peanut is *cacahouète*. This method also works well in ethnic restaurants in the United States and may also come in handy if you need to seek emergency medical treatment when the practitioner is not fluent in English.

Montezuma's Revenge

Gastrointestinal infections can result from drinking contaminated water or eating uncooked or improperly cooked foods. Any raw food could be contaminated, particularly in areas of poor sanitation. In addition to the allergens you always want to avoid, you must be aware of additional foods that could cause further complications. Of special concern are salads, uncooked vegetables and fruit, raw meat, and shellfish.

Some fish aren't guaranteed safe even when cooked, because of the presence of toxins in their flesh. Tropical reef fish, red snapper, amber jack, grouper, and sea bass may be toxic if they're caught on tropical reefs rather than in open ocean. Highest-risk areas include the islands of the West Indies and the tropical Pacific and Indian Oceans.

Typical symptoms of what is popularly known, particularly in Mexico and Central America, as Montezuma's Revenge, are diarrhea, nausea, fever, and bloating. The condition can be caused by viruses, bacteria, or parasites that contaminate food or water. High-risk areas include the developing countries of Africa, the Middle East, Mexico, and Central America.

An antibiotic such as Cipro or Noroxin, combined with Immodium AD tablets, will treat most cases.

Timely Tip

Health-care facilities in your destination country may not be as good as what you have at home, particularly in third-world countries. If you're taking an adventure holiday, make sure adequate facilities are available should you need urgent treatment. Contact the tour operator well ahead of time to start your due diligence. This way, you'll learn what you have to do to make sure you're covered.

Beyond Our Borders

Reports of food allergies began to appear in Europe in the early 1900s, and since the 1940s, food allergies have been recognized by doctors around the world.

Some 1,800 restaurant outlets across Canada, including 9 national chains, are now participating in Allergy Aware, a program that provides diners with information on common allergens in restaurant menu items. Look for the Allergy Aware symbol in restaurant windows.

Look for this symbol for safe dining across Canada.

The Assurance of Insurance

In foreign countries, many American insurance plans are invalid. So before you leave on your trip abroad, find out what medical services, if any, your health insurance will cover. If your policy does provide coverage overseas, remember to carry your insurance ID card as proof, together with a claim form. Although many companies will pay "customary and reasonable" hospital costs abroad, very few will pay for your medical evacuation back to the United States. Medical evacuation can cost $10,000 and up, depending on your location and medical condition.

Hospitals abroad often require a substantial cash deposit. A variety of travel insurance plans, including some that arrange for emergency evacuation, are available through travel agents and some credit card companies.

The Social Security Medicare program does not provide coverage for hospital or medical costs outside the United States. Senior citizens may contact the American Association of Retired Persons (AARP) for information about foreign medical care coverage with Medicare supplement plans. (For more contact information, see Appendix B.)

Consult Your Consul

In case of illness, American citizens traveling overseas should know about the services offered by U.S. embassies and consulates. United States consulates may help secure emergency medical services. Consular officers can assist in transferring funds and informing relatives of a health condition; however, they cannot act as lawyers or bankers, and payment of hospital and other expenses is the responsibility of the traveler.

A list of addresses and telephone numbers of U.S. embassies and consulates may be obtained through the Superintendent of Documents, U.S. Government Printing Office, Washington, DC 20402. Names of reliable English-speaking doctors worldwide are available from several travel organizations. U.S. embassies and consulates abroad maintain lists of hospitals and physicians. Major credit card companies also can provide the names of local doctors and hospitals abroad. For contact information, please refer to Appendix B.

Last-Minute Wrap-Ups

Here are a few travel items you won't want to forget:

- ◆ When traveling out of the country, carry a letter from your physician describing your medical condition and listing prescription medications, including the generic names of prescribed drugs. Medications should be left in their original containers and be clearly labeled.

- ◆ Check with the foreign embassies of the countries you're visiting to make sure your required medications are not considered illegal narcotics.

- ◆ Be sure to carry a doctor's note if you carry an EpiPen. After September 11, an EpiPen might be considered a weapon by some of the more scrupulous inspectors.

- ◆ Write a short letter indicating that you have a serious food allergy and listing the foods and ingredients, including hidden ingredients, you must avoid at all costs, and have it translated into the language of your destination. If you don't feel comfortable communicating your allergy problem and special food requests to the staff in European restaurants because of a language barrier, pull out the letter and show it to the staff. For your convenience, we have provided such a letter in five languages that you may wish to use.

Letters to Live (and Eat) By

If you don't feel comfortable communicating your allergy problem and special food requests to European restaurants because of a language barrier, you may want to copy the following letter, which we've translated into French, Italian, Spanish, and German for your convenience, and edit it to reflect your particular allergy problems, so you can present it at the various restaurants you frequent abroad. English, first.

To Whom It May Concern

To Whom It May Concern:

I have a serious food allergy which I would like to bring to your attention. It is important that the foods you serve me do not contain any of the following ingredients, including hidden ingredients:

Dairy products (milk, cheese, yogurt, etc.), eggs, fish, shellfish (lobster, clams, oysters, etc.), tree nuts (walnuts, almonds, etc.), peanuts, soy, wheat, citrus, chocolate, strawberries.

If I should mistakenly eat even a small amount of the food to which I am allergic, I could become gravely ill and perhaps even die.

Thank you for your help.

Ciao, Italia–Mangia, Mangia!

Attenzione, per piacere:

Sono allergico(a) agli alimenti elencati sotto. È importante che i cibi che voi mi servete non contienanno alcuni degli ingredienti, perfino ingredienti nascosti, elen-catti sotto:

> Prodotti del caseificio (il latte, il formaggio, il yogurt ecc.), le uove, il pesce, il mollusco (l'aragosta, le vongole, l'ostriche, ecc.), i noci raccoglie dagli alberi, le noccioline, la soia, il grano, l'arancio, il cioccolato, le fragole.

Se mangio sbagliatamente anche una piccola quantità del cibo al quale sono allergico (allergica), potrei divenire gravemente malato (malata), e forse potrei perfino morire.

Grazie per il vostro aiuto.

Bon Voyage et Bon Appétit–J'aime la France

Attention, s'il vous plaît:

Je suis allergique á certains produits alimentaires. Il est impératif que les plats que vous me serviez ne contiennent pas les ingrédients ci-dessous (même en forme cachée):

> De produits laitiers (de lait, de fromage, de yaourt, etc.), d'oeufs, de poisson, de crustacés (de homard, de palourdes, d'huîtres, etc.), de noix des arbres, de caca-houètes, de soja, de blé, d'oranges, de pamplemousse, de mandarines, de choco-lat, de fraises.

Si j'en mangeais même une petite quan-tité, je pourrais devenir gravement malade et je pourrais même mourir.

Je vous remercie.

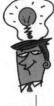

Bet You Didn't Know _____

In Spanish, the word for peanut is *cacahuete*; the word for peanut butter is *manteca de cacahuete* or *manilla*; for peanut oil: *aceite de cacahuete*. In most parts of Spain and South America, they frequently use the word *frutas secas* (dried fruits), when referring to nuts. However, in both Spain and Latin America the word *nuez* (nut) is also used.

Ole! Mucho Gusto!

Atención, por favor:

Soy muy alérgico(a) a ciertas comestibles. Y es imperativo que mis comidas no contengan los ingredientes siguientes, incluyendo ingredientes ocultos:

> Productos lácteos (leche, queso, yogur, etc.), huevos, pez, mariscos (langostas, almejas, ostras, etc.), árbol chiflado (nueces, almendras, etc.), cacahuetes, soja, trigo, cítricos, chocolate, fresas.

Si yo comiera una cantidad pequeña de ciertos comestibles podría ponerme gravemente enfermo y quizás podría morirme.

Gracias por su ayuda.

Delicatessen, Über Alles

Ich bitte um Ihre Aufmerksamkeit:

Ich habe eine ernstzunehmende Speiseallergie auf die ich Sie hinweisen möchte. Es ist wichtig, dass die Mahlzeiten die Sie mir servieren, unter keinen Umständen auch nur eine der folgenden Zutaten enthalten (auch nicht in versteckter Form):

> Molkerei Produkte, Eier, Schalentiere, Baumnüsse, Erdnüsse, Sojabohnen, Zitrusfrüchte, Schokolade, Erdbeeren

Sollte ich auch nur versehentlich etwas essen das diese Zutaten enthält, könnte ich ernsthaft krank werden.

Herzlichen Dank für Ihr Verständnis.

The Least You Need to Know

- Dining in restaurants is the most difficult aspect of having a food allergy.
- Safe dining is possible, but considerable preparation and detective work are necessary.
- Nut and peanut allergies are especially dangerous for allergic diners, because many dishes have hidden ingredients.
- It is possible to enjoy travel despite a food allergy.

Part 5

Alternative and Complementary Help

Alternative and complementary treatments for food allergy offer a vast array of options, from acupuncture and acupressure to shiatsu and yoga. However, beware that not all the treatments and therapies discussed in this part are what they are made out to be by their practitioners.

Note: The information and content in this part are only for the general information of the reader and should not be relied on as medical advice. No endorsement, opinion, or other recommendation is offered by the authors or the publisher with respect to the information provided herein. The theories of treatment discussed herein are not to be considered alternative forms of therapy or treatment, and are not recognized by conventional medical caregivers, including medical physicians, doctors of osteopathy, or nurse practitioners. The reader is strongly encouraged to seek out his or her own trained medical practitioner for advice, diagnosis, and treatment regarding any medical condition.

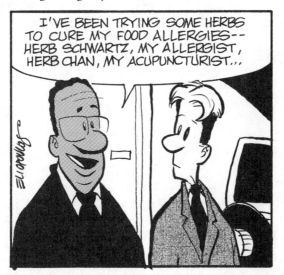

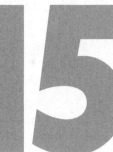

Quackery, Thy Name Is Legion

In This Chapter

- Learn to spot charlatans who promote phony cures
- Understand the facts about environmental disease and multiple chemical sensitivity
- Learn about useless, unsound allergy tests
- Discover why alternative and complementary medicines are popular

More and more Americans are entrusting their health care to practitioners of alternative medicine, who specialize in relaxation techniques, chiropractic treatments, herbal medicines, massages, acupuncture, aromatherapy, biofeedback, naturopathy, reflexology, yoga, and other alternative therapies. Although many of these treatments may help patients with some of their problems—especially when used in conjunction with conventional medical treatments—the field of alternative medicine is wide open for abuse by unqualified individuals with over-hyped modalities and "cures"—many of which not only lack scientific proof, but can be dangerous to the health of the patient.

According to the *New England Journal of Medicine*, one third of American adults seek unorthodox therapy annually, while the FDA reports that nearly 40 million Americans have used fraudulent health remedies within the past year, and that Americans spend close to $30 billion per year on quack health products and treatments. This chapter provides an overview of those quack modalities that claim to diagnose, treat, and even cure food allergy.

Profiles in Deception

Alternative practitioners rarely undertake scientific studies of illnesses. In fact, many such people disdain science. You should be aware that there are many false diagnostic methods and spurious follow-up recommendations proposed by some alternative practitioners. From patients heeding improper advice, potentially life-threatening problems have occurred, including nerve damage and allergic reactions. In fact, one out of every ten people who try quack remedies is harmed by the side effects, while one in ten doctors report serious side effects triggered by unorthodox methods. Incorrect diagnoses cause patients unnecessary worry and waste their time and money. Worse, when patients commit themselves to a bogus therapy, they risk ignoring a potentially valid scientific treatment that could help their condition, warns Stephen Barrett, M.D., a practicing Pennsylvania physician whose website, www.quackwatch.com, cautions readers against bogus alternative therapies.

Bet You Didn't Know

Health practices are called alternative if they are based on untested or unscientific principles. If an alternative health treatment is followed in tandem with conventional medicine, it is referred to as complementary medicine. While many of the practices in this area have been examined by mainstream medicine and received acknowledgment as being useful, others are pure quackery, with no scientific evidence to support them.

Fad Diagnoses

Some practitioners, whose qualifications may range from well-meaning but misinformed to out-and-out fraudsters, are diagnosing "food allergy" in patients via methods not recognized by the scientific community.

A few current fad diagnoses touted by these practitioners that are often used to explain alleged or real allergy symptoms are environmental illness, multiple chemical sensitivity, leaky gut syndrome, mercury amalgam toxicity, and Wilson's Syndrome. The latter was invented by a debunked Florida doctor, who claims that his syndrome can cause "virtually every symptom known to man," including, of course, food allergies. (Although

Wilson's Syndrome is a bogus diagnosis, there is a valid condition known as Wilson's Disease, a rare condition caused by a defect in the body's ability to metabolize copper, as explained in Chapter 5.)

Food Allergy—Disease *du Jour*

If you have a real food allergy, you're right in vogue, because food allergy has the distinction of having become the twenty-first century fad diagnosis, the current hip disease *du jour*. Added to this, 25 percent of the population believes they have a food allergy when they actually do not. Capitalizing on this dubious craze, a parade of charlatans has come out of the woodwork to "diagnose" food allergies in patients, even where they do not exist. In some cases, patients who are not food allergic are wrongly diagnosed, when they are actually suffering from other conditions.

Patients with troublesome symptoms are often diagnosed with environmental illness (EI), also labeled multiple chemical sensitivity (MCS). In this condition, it is said that when the total load of physical stress exceeds a person's toleration level, the immune system goes berserk, causing hypersensitivity to tiny amounts of foods and chemicals to trigger a range of unpleasant symptoms.

Doctors advocating the EI/MCS theory call themselves clinical ecologists, or specialists in environmental medicine. The American Academy of Allergy, Asthma and Immunology (AAAAI), the nation's largest professional organization of allergists, warns that "a causal connection between environmental chemicals, foods, and/or drugs and the patient's symptoms is speculative and not based on the results of published scientific studies."

Clinical ecologists chiefly base their diagnoses on provocation and neutralization tests, which are performed by having the patient report symptoms that occur within ten minutes after suspected substances are administered under the tongue or injected into the skin. Researchers at the University of California have demonstrated that such procedures are invalid.

Tests That Don't Make the Cut

An ever-increasing number of bogus practitioners claim that food allergies are responsible for virtually any and every symptom in existence, from chronic fatigue to obesity. In support of their false claims, they administer various screening and evaluation methods purported to pinpoint the foods responsible for hidden allergies. Here is a list of the dubious allergy tests you don't want to take:

- **ALCAT.** The test supposedly measures how blood cells react to foods under conditions designed to mimic "what happens when the foods are consumed in real life." Contrary to claims, the test does not accurately test for food allergies.

- **Applied Kinesiology (AK).** The patient's arm strength and muscle weakness are tested when exposed to allergens held in a glass vial in front of a magnetic field. Double-blind studies have found no benefit from this technique. (A double-blind test is a control-group test where neither the evaluator nor the subject knows which items are controls. The double refers to the fact the food is given in a disguised form, such as a gelatin capsule, and a placebo nonactive material is given in exactly the same capsules. Each is numbered with a code number. The reactions are noted and recorded. No one knows the contents of the capsules until after the test is completed and the code is broken.)

Skulls and Bones _____

Don't waste your time and money on biocranial technique (BCT) or adrenal gland tests. They cannot diagnose food allergies.

- **Auriculo-cardiac reflex.** Suspected allergens are placed in filter papers on the arm. A bright light is shone through the ear lobe or hand, while the pulse is taken to check for increases. No scientific data has validated this test.

- **Bryan's leucocytotoxic test.** This test is a variation of the leucocytotoxic test (see later in this list). When the patient's white blood cells are mixed with allergens, the blood cells swell. The tests then measure the swelling to determine how much allergen must be added to damage the cells.

- **Cytotoxic tests.** These tests involve taking a blood sample, extracting the white blood cells, and exposing them to suspected food allergens on slides. Proponents of these tests believe that if the patient is allergic to a particular food it will affect the white blood cells, and these changes can be observed under a microscope. However, the results of these tests are largely inconsistent. There is hope, though, that someday cytotoxic tests might be of some value if results can be reproduced consistently under carefully controlled conditions. At this time, however, commercial cytotoxic tests are of very little value. Yet, proponents use the results to explain symptoms and to design a "personalized diet program" that includes vitamins and minerals (sold by those administering the test).

- **Desensitization.** In this test, progressively larger doses of a food are injected to determine an allergy. (This technique may work for allergies related to inhaled substances, but does not for food allergy, and can be dangerous.)

- **ELISA/ACT.** This test was developed by Russell Jaffe, M.D., Ph.D., performed by Jaffe's Serammune Physicians Lab (SPL), of Reston, Virginia. ELISA/ACT's brochure states that as much as 60 percent of all illness is due to hidden allergies. Their test cultures the patient's lymphocytes to determine reactions to up to 300 foods. They also recommend supplements to overcome the allergy. There is no evidence to suggest this test has any diagnostic value. (Do not confuse the ELISA/ACT test with the ELISA test, which is a recognized test for some infectious diseases, a variation of which is used for food allergy testing.)

- **Hair analysis.** Hair is made up of a protein of keratin. This can be analyzed to determine the mineral content of the hair, which in turn can be used to find out if the body is lacking in certain minerals. That's it! According to proponents of this testing method, mineral content of the hair is supposedly related to food allergies. Double-blind studies have failed to show diagnostic value to this test.

- **IgG blood tests.** These tests are conducted by practitioners who believe that delayed food allergies are mediated by IgG antibodies. However, there is no foundation for these claims. Although IgG levels can be raised in food sensitivity, they are not related to any particular food problem. In other words, if you are sensitive to eggs your IgG to eggs may be raised, but so may be your IgG to other foods. Conventional allergists suspect that this can be traced to a leaky gut, which permits more food antigens to pass into the bloodstream.

- **Leucocytotoxic test.** The patient's white blood cells are mixed with allergens to detect cell damage. A high number of false positive and negative reactions led the American Academy of Allergy to declare there is no benefit to these tests.

- **Live cell microscopy.** Used by the chiropractic community and other practitioners, this device, despite claims, has no scientific application in detecting allergies.

- **N.A.E.T. (Nambudripad's Allergy Elimination Technique).** A system of diagnosis and treatment based on the concept that allergies are caused by "energy blockage" that can be diagnosed with muscle-testing, and permanently cured with acupressure and/or acupuncture.

- **Neutralization.** Progressively smaller food doses are administered until the patient no longer reacts to them. No value has been found in this procedure.

- **NuTron testing.** Claims to measure the reactivity of white blood cells to food and other substances, then designs a diet eliminating foods causing "white blood cell activation." Adherents say the proposed diet will improve conditions caused by the release of "inflammatory chemicals from the activated white cells." In over 40 years, no studies have ever shown the test to be accurate.

- **Provocation neutralization tests.** In these tests the suspected food is put under the patient's tongue or injected in increasing doses under the first layer of skin. The patient is then observed for subtle signs of an allergy such as perspiration, feeling funny, and nonmeasurable changes reported by the patient. No diagnostic reliability has been found for this test.

- **Pulse tests.** Advocates of these tests claim that a patient's pulse rate increases markedly after the intake of allergy-causing foods. Most conventional allergists maintain, however, that there may be other reasons for this occurrence and a rising pulse rate by itself is not enough to make a valid diagnosis.

- **Sublingual testing.** Suspected foods are placed under the tongue for analysis.

- **The LEAP Program.** Uses the Mediator Release Test (MRT) to identify putative delayed food allergies. Recommended treatment then consists of dietary changes, supplements, and herbs.

Risky Risk Management

Alternative and complementary medicines not only produce questionable views of allergy testing, they also purport to treat food allergies in various ways that do not work and could be dangerous. Here are a few modalities to avoid:

- **Enzyme potentiated desensitization.** This treatment involves mixing allergens with beta-glucuronidase, an enzyme in the body, and applying it to the skin in low doses. Double-blind studies have failed to show any significant benefit using this regimen.

- **Ionization.** You've seen them advertised on TV. Negative ion machines emit negative electric charges into the air and have been claimed to help hay fever and asthma sufferers by decreasing the allergen load on the nasal mucosa and lungs; however, there are no studies available to substantiate this claim.

- **Speleotherapy.** Also known as underground climatotherapy, this is an alternative treatment for asthma that involves spending 2 to 3 hours a day underground in subterranean caves or salt mines over a 2- to 3-month period. This is an old therapeutic modality without a scientific explanation.

- **Ozone therapy.** Proponents advocate that the allergic patient's blood be exposed to ozone gas, then ozone be infused rectally or vaginally. This practice could have serious adverse results.

Iridology: Tale of the Iris

Iridology, also known as iris diagnosis, is yet another in a long list of methods that purport to diagnose food allergies (in addition to a host of other conditions).

This practice is based on the concept that each part of the body is represented by a corresponding area in the iris of the eye, and that health conditions can be determined from examining the eye's color and texture, as well as the location of various pigment flecks. Iridologists claim they diagnose body imbalances that will then be treated with vitamins, minerals, homeopathic remedies, and herbs, which they recommend and sell to the client.

Some iridologists also claim that eye markings reveal a complete history of past illnesses, including surgeries. For instance, a white triangle in a certain area indicates appendicitis, whereas a black speck indicates the appendix has been removed.

Iridology as a system of diagnosis is said to have been invented by nineteenth-century Hungarian physician Ignatz von Peczely, who, in childhood, after accidentally breaking the leg of an owl noticed a black stripe in the lower part of the owl's eye that gradually changed to a white ("healing") line as the owl's leg healed. Upon his release from prison following the Hungarian Revolution of 1848, von Peczely, recalling the long-ago incident of the owl's eye, began studying the eyes of his patients, and also performed many autopsies, experiences through which he devised the iridology diagnostic system.

Med Meaning

Iridology is the study of the iris of the eye, the exposed nerve endings that are connected to the brain. It is said that a trained iridologist can tell genetic inheritance, congestive, and irritative zones and their various inter-reactions within the body. Thus, iridology provides information needed to establish the root cause of ailments and reveals appropriate treatments required.

Parting of the Ways

Mainstream physicians describe the iris as the part of the eye that regulates light. At the center of the iris is a contractile opening, the pupil, which admits light to the lens. The lens in turn brings light rays into focus, forming images upon the retina, where light falls upon rods and cones, causing them to stimulate the optic nerve, which transmits visual impressions to the brain.

Iridologists maintain that neuro-optic reflexed information, provided by more than 28,000 exposed nerve endings, links the iris to the body via the sympathetic nervous system. The iris is made up of connective tissue containing thousands of nerve endings, all of which are connected to the brain. Iridologists say that each organ has a counterpart in the eye and that through an iris exam, troubled areas receiving "referred symptoms" are also identified. For example, most heart problems, say iridologists, are first caused by trouble in the descending colon. This, iridology says, comes from information that developed with the embryo, and is connected with the electrical system of the body. The brain receives continual information regarding organ function and records these messages in iris markings. In this way iridology identifies and treats health issues.

Skulls and Bones

There is no known mechanism by which body organs can be represented or transmit their health status to specific locations in the iris.

Skulls and Bones

Some multilevel distributors use iridology as a basis for recommending dietary supplements and herbs. Anyone who does this and is not a licensed health professional would be guilty of practicing medicine without a license.

While traditional physicians recognize that some symptoms of nonocular conditions can be detected by an eye exam, and that the eyes may change appearance when certain health conditions are present, medical science says there is no evidence showing that the iris is connected to any of the body's organs.

Iridologists, however, believe the iris is divided into 40 zones, each corresponding to different body parts. By looking at a particular part of the iris, iridologists say they can identify warning signs, through abnormal spots, colors, or lines. The nerve endings of each iris respond through the spinal cord, optic ganglia, and optic nerves to all parts of the body. The iris lines, flecks, and pigments guide the iridologist not only to what is wrong at examination time, but also to what was wrong in the past or what could go wrong in the future.

Where's the Proof?

Published studies report no evidence in support of a functional iris-body connection, including studies conducted by the University of California at San Diego and the University of Melbourne, Australia. Further, iridologists themselves disagree on patient diagnosis. Their iris evaluations are made based on 20 or more different iris charts. One former iridologist even gave up practicing after examining Polaroid films of a number of his patients and finding out that although their symptoms had improved, their eye markings had not. Given the track record, many have had no choice but to dub iridology a pseudo-science.

Still, many of iridology's more than 10,000 practitioners worldwide use iridology to diagnose food allergies.

Bet You Didn't Know

The diagnostic method of sclerology, which was developed by Native Americans, is similar to iridology but interprets the shape and condition of blood vessels on the white portion (sclera) of the eyeball.

Taking a Peek at the "P" Cure

A glass a day keeps the doctor away, say advocates of the "P" cure. That's right, "P" as in pee, otherwise known as urine. Drinking your own urine is said by millions worldwide to be good for what ails you. It's a miracle cure with untold benefits, say its proponents. Of course, it is considered by its advocates to cure food allergies—and more. In fact, many advocates claim there is practically nothing urine won't cure. It is said to be effective against skin problems, and is helpful with allergies, constipation, eczema, eye irritation, immunological disorders, urticaria, congestion, gastritis, and more. It is even claimed that asthma can be cured with auto urine therapy.

The Historical Background of the "P" Cure

The origin of this unusual practice can be traced to ancient Hindu religious rites, where it is called *amaroli* in tantric tradition. Indian yogis reportedly have been drinking their own urine for over 5,000 years. In the "Vedas," sacred Hindu writings, it is said that the nectar of the gods, called *amrita*, beverage of immortality, is urine.

In China, according to the Chinese pharmaceutical dictionary *Shang Han Lun*, urine was traditionally used as a medium for delivery of medicinal herbs to strengthen their effects. It has been reported that Indian yogis as well as lamas of Tibet reached extended ages by drinking their own urine.

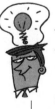

Bet You Didn't Know

Two famous books on urine therapy are the 1918 classic *Urine as an Autotherapeutic Remedy*, by Dr. Charles H. Duncan, followed by John W. Armstrong's *The Water of Life*, published in 1944.

Drinking urine for therapeutic purposes also was practiced en masse in the Holy Roman Empire, when urinal troughs were erected in the public squares of each city-state for residents to both contribute to and benefit from. In ancient Rome, urine was so important that the emperor placed a tax on every drop.

Bet You Didn't Know

The Miracle Cup of Liquid Institute, Japan, founded by Dr. Ryoichi Nakao, is an organization for people practicing urine therapy. The institute was founded to help the estimated two million urine therapy advocates in Japan, as well as to help spread urine therapy around the world.

The Age of Reason

In the eighteenth century, Europeans used not only human urine, but also cow urine, to build up and maintain health, and especially to cure asthma. In the early 1800s, a book titled *One Thousand Notable Things* describes the use of urine to relieve skin itching and many other conditions.

In more modern times, the Alaskan Eskimos and European Gypsies are known to be advocates of this therapy.

Urine Immunity?

Although some toxic substances could be present, especially if one is ill, urine is a non-toxic substance. The small amount of urine's toxic substances, it is said, contributes to the effectiveness of urine therapy. If toxic substances enter the body, the body's defense mechanisms are called into action. A similar process takes place with vaccination. This stimulates the immune system to manufacture antibodies to defend the body.

One expert suggests that the presence of antigens and antibodies in urine strengthens the immune system when urine is reintroduced into the body; small amounts of bacteria or parasites found in urine may stimulate the production of IgE, which prevents micro-organisms from becoming embedded in the mucous.

Most advocates prefer to drink their morning discharge. Some prefer it straight; others mix it with orange juice or serve it over fruit or cereal. Some devotees use their own urine as an enema; others wash themselves in the golden liquid to improve skin quality. Many modern Japanese women engage in urine bathing. (There is no report on the reaction of the men in their lives.)

The main attractions of "P" therapy are cost and availability. The main danger is that the urine contains protein from the person's body. The immune system does not know that, especially if the urine should be given by injection. The immune system identifies this protein as foreign or nonself. Next it creates antibodies against this protein, which is the person's own kidneys. Thus is created autoimmune kidney disease, kidney failure, and dialysis leading to transplant. Not a pretty picture. This is more common with injection therapy than drinking the urine because the GI tract would not allow the protein through and into the bloodstream.

 Skulls and Bones

The Chinese Association of Urine Therapy warns that not everybody can just start right in drinking their own urine without some negative side effects. It will take some getting used to.

Meeting the "Magic" of Magnets

Magnets have been used for pain for centuries, and have been increasing as a fad in the United States. Magnets, it is said by the products' promoters, have no side effects, at least none yet revealed, and at the same time the cost is minimal, making them seem, for some people, an attractive adjunctive therapy. But is this really so?

Magnets usually come encased in a wrap, which is placed about the head or neck for periods of time ranging from minutes to hours. Some people sleep on a magnet pillow, or on a bed with a mattress pad lined with magnets. You can purchase magnets from any number of different companies that make these products in an amazing number of different forms. Department stores, pharmacies, health food stores, catalog houses, the Internet, and many other types of retail outlets can supply any size or shape magnet you desire. But wait … before you throw your money away, are you sure you really want to use magnets?

Magnets are a very touchy subject; they have become a major scam in Southern California and other places, involving both hucksters and doctors trying to make an extra buck. A leading California allergist got taken, as did several of his neighbors, by a local sales pitch with a guaranteed money back offer. "Chronic pain leads one to do dumb things," admits this physician, who has asked that his name be withheld. The doctor goes on to say:

Skulls and Bones

Magnets shouldn't be used if you have a cardiac pacemaker or other internal device. They also should not be used if pregnancy is possible. Better yet, save your money and don't use them at all.

> I practice in an area of the state which is horse country, and many of my nurses have horses. They use magnets on the horses' legs for sprains and joint problems. So I figured if it's good enough for a horse, it's good enough for me. A thousand dollars later, I discover the magnets are not doing any good at all—not the mattress, not the neck piece or anything else I was gullible enough to buy from

these scamsters. So what about that money back guarantee? Turns out every company and sales office has closed up and left town, or changed its name and telephone number. As you might expect, if the fraud division of the local and federal authorities ever catches up to these people, they face a long stretch in jail. Since I and many out there were scammed, there have been public announcements warning the general public about this.

New Waves from over the Ocean

To do some thinking out of the box, let's explore the controversial field of bio-energetic testing—a technique that has been used for decades on several continents throughout the world but has gone largely unrecognized in North America.

The idea that the body is charged with energy that can be measured quantitatively with a specialized device is nothing new; the electrocardiogram (EKG) is used as a clinical tool in the diagnosis of heart disease. Unlike the EKG, however, machines that purport to discover (and even recommend treatment for) food allergies by testing body energy have yet to convince the medical establishment in the United States and Canada of their merits.

The Origin of the Species

Electrodermal screening (EDS), also known as *electrodermal testing* (EDT), is a method of allergy testing that originated with a diagnostic procedure known as *Electro-Acupuncture According to Voll* (EAV), an invention of German physician Reinhold Voll.

Med Meaning

Electrodermal screening/ testing (EDS/EDT) is an unorthodox technique to diagnose allergies and other diseases. Unlike traditional skin-prick allergy tests, EDS/EDT is said to rely on imbalances in the body's electrical circuit instead of the body's immune system to test for food allergies.

Dr. Voll was an orthodox physician as well as a homeopath who studied Chinese medicine and acupuncture. He combined all three theories with galvanic skin differentials to produce his technique.

In the 1970s, Dr. William Tiller, Stanford University Professor of Physics (now Emeritus), verified that the skin displays unique electrical reactions to various impulses, especially over acupuncture points. His research shed more light on the interplay between mind, body, and subtle energies. He is credited with further developing Dr. Voll's work.

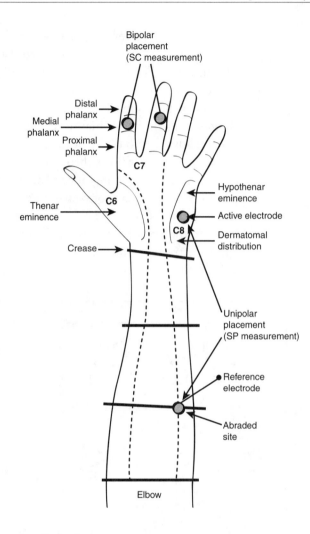

Proponents of EDS/EDT say the body's acupuncture points have an electrical resistance from which it's possible to pinpoint disturbances, including food allergies.

Measuring Mind and Matter

Proponents allege that EDS/EDT devices can help people suffering from such food allergy symptoms as bloating, irritable bowel syndrome, skin rashes, pain, inflammatory disorders, and disturbances such as asthma, bronchitis, and gastritis. They also claim to be able to identify early precursors to disease.

So suppose you decide to be tested with an EDS/EDT machine. What can you expect? Relax, this testing is simple and painless. You will sit in a comfortable chair, take your shoes off, and be prepared to spend a very short time being tested, probably between three minutes and a half-hour at most, depending on which manufacturer's machine your operator is using.

Bet You Didn't Know _____

Varieties of electrodermal testing machines, with slight variations, are currently used by several hundred thousand medical doctors in Europe, Asia, Australia, and the Middle East, as well as by several thousand holistic health advocates in the United States and Canada—even though some FDA restrictions on the technique exist.

Actual testing involves measuring electromagnetic conductivity in your body, using a Wheatstone bridge galvanometer. The machine operator will place one electrode over your acupuncture points, while another electrode will be applied to a battery of selected allergens and chemicals that have been placed in a metallic honeycomb of the device. The machine emits a current that flows through a wire to the probe you are holding in your hand, and measures the electrical resistance of your skin when contacted by the probe. Energy and information flow from the device to the probe and back. A change in the reading of electromagnetic conductivity is believed to indicate allergy or intolerance to that allergen.

EDT devices are designed to detect whether someone is allergic or sensitive to foods.

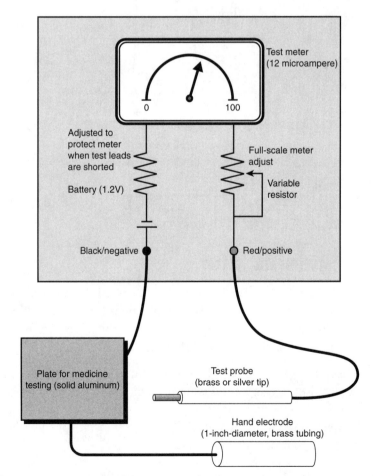

Claims and Counterclaims

Although physicians are enthusiastic users of this technique in other parts of the world, EDT has not caught on with doctors in the United States and Canada. In fact, most physicians here have never even heard of it. If you're seeking a knowledgeable professional to administer the method in North America, you might, if you persist, find a holistic physician practitioner or environmental medicine physician; allergist proponents, few and far between, are harder to find. The most visible EDT advocates comprise a coterie of acupuncturists, naturopaths, homeopaths, herbologists, chiropractors, dieticians, dentists, veterinarians, and nutritionists, who swear by the technique. In fact, you may have seen EDS promoters, together with their equipment, in shopping malls and health food markets; at booths in health expos and trade shows; or in space rented at flea markets, without even realizing what they were doing.

In some instances, advocates' assertions have been challenged by federal and state regulatory agencies. The FDA, which regulates medical devices in the United States, classifies "devices that use resistance measurements to diagnose and treat allergy" as Class III devices, which require approval before they can be legally used. Following this, the machines may then be marketed on an "investigation only" basis.

The manufacturer's literature must state that if the machine is used for medical diagnosis, it must bear the label "For investigation use only. The performance characteristics of this product have not been established," and that any diagnosis must be confirmed by an accepted medical procedure, such as a RAST test. Even so, prohibitions are not strictly enforced, and most device operators know that authorities cannot police every instance in every city and town.

Outlawed but Omnipresent

Although detractors insist there are no controlled studies to support EDS/EDT claims, proponents point to many trials in Europe and Asia; Russian, Czech, Chinese, and other studies have cited the efficacy of the technique. Not long ago, the validity of electrodermal testing was challenged by a study in the British Medical Journal. Although the Journal questioned EDS/EDT's effectiveness for diagnosing allergies to cat dander and dust mites, it agreed that perhaps the method was useful for diagnosing food sensitivities.

The Art of Spotting Quackery

If you are tempted to believe the claims of borderline and dubious practitioners who say they can cure your health problems, remember, there is no "cure" for food allergies.

Your allergy may possibly vanish, but more than likely, it will not. In any case, do not expect alternative medical miracles from charlatan promoters purporting to have all the answers.

Few scientific studies are done by "alternative" practitioners. If you are confronted with a purported "cure," be wary—especially if the "evidence" consists merely of testimonials, self-published material, or paid-for advertising.

Big Business, Big Bucks

Why does borderline alternative health care continue to be so popular? Here are some of the reasons:

◆ Fear of surgery and drugs alienate many people from conventional medicine, leading them to an alternative practice because its treatments are noninvasive.

◆ The risks of being harmed by an alternative practitioner are thought to be less than by a conventional physician who prescribes drugs and performs surgery.

◆ Alternative medicine is thought to be using "natural" remedies. Many people erroneously believe that what is natural is better and safer than pharmaceutical drugs.

◆ Alternative medicine has emotional appeal and a mystical quality. It provides hope, even when the situation is hopeless.

◆ Alternative treatment is usually less expensive than conventional medicine.

◆ People believe alternative health care works; they feel better and may even think they're cured.

Cure or Curse? Buyer Beware!

Far too many questionable modalities touted as effective are pure quackery. Watch out if:

◆ Text is written in impressive-sounding terminology that disguises a lack of underlying science.

◆ A promoter claims "the system" (government, medical profession, multinational drug companies, and so on) has conspired to suppress his method or product.

◆ The modality is advertised as available from only one source.

◆ The promoter uses words such as scientific breakthrough, miraculous cure, secret ingredient, or ancient remedy.

Another thing to keep in mind: Results of studies on bona fide treatments are reported first in medical journals after passing peer review. If promotions for a treatment appear via other means, it's probably because the treatment can't pass scientific trials.

The general rule to follow is: "If it sounds too good to be true, it probably is."

The Least You Need to Know

♦ Many unorthodox, unproven, and fraudulent methods purport to diagnose allergies, but they do not.

♦ Quacksters, fraudsters, and other charlatans prey upon the vulnerable allergy patient.

♦ With the immense popularity of alternative therapies, the allergy patient must be wary of incompetent practitioners.

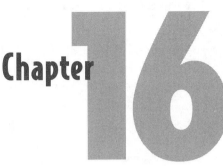
A Visit to the Health Food Store

In This Chapter

- ◆ Discover herbs that may help allergic symptoms
- ◆ Learn what vitamins, minerals, and supplements can complement your allergy treatment
- ◆ Find out how aromatherapy and essential oils may soothe your allergy symptoms

As people are taking responsibility for their own health, they are reaching out in growing numbers to alternative and complementary medicine. Some individuals, including those with food allergies, have even opted out of mainstream medicine altogether in favor of herbal cures, vitamins, and supplements to regulate their problems. While some people have undertaken a reasonable study of the vast, complex field of herbology and vitamins/supplements, others are going merely on trust when they pick up a product at their local health food store or supermarket or place an order from the Internet.

If you want to take herbs for relief of symptoms caused by a food allergy, vitamins that may complement your food allergy medical treatment, or if you wish to consider the possibility of essential oils and aromatherapy providing benefits in soothing bothersome food allergy symptoms, there are facts you should know before you buy and try. At the very least, you should be aware of the pros and cons. But first, a disclaimer: We do not advocate you opt out of mainstream medicine in favor of herbal or vitamin solutions to your food allergy problem. This chapter should be read for information only, after which we strongly recommend you consult your allergist before trying any of the listed items.

The Power of Pills

Modern pharmacy owes a great deal to herbs. Aspirin's origin is found in willow bark, atropine comes from belladonna, which is found in the deadly nightshade plant, and morphine originates in poppies, to mention a few examples. But if plants' benefits are manifold, so are their dangers. When herbs from plants are marketed, they are frequently said to be "natural." Most people assume this means they're safe; however, such may not be the case.

Natural Dangers

Many people with food allergies experience asthmatic attacks. One much-hyped herb used by food allergic asthmatics has been a particularly egregious offender. Ephedra, also known as ephedrine and Ma Huang, which causes rising blood pressure and increased heart rate, has also been known to cause significant nerve and muscle damage, memory loss, stroke, psychosis, and even death. Despite the fact that the Food and Drug Administration (FDA) has issued many warnings concerning this herb and recommended limiting its levels in health food products, some supplements on the shelves still contain far more than the FDA recommended amount. Other dangers of using this herb include interaction with other medication, with detrimental effects.

If you have a food allergy and decide you want to try herbs for relief of symptoms, the use of herbal supplements must be done with caution. Before using any supplements, discuss the matter with your physician, and be sure the herbs you want to take are appropriate for your medical needs. The amount of therapeutic drugs found in herbs in their raw state varies greatly from plant to plant, root to root, and even leaf to leaf. Added to this, many of the herbs used in capsules are imported from Asia, where controls are lax, and have proven dangerous to the consumer.

What's in an Herb?

Herbs come in many different forms: dried roots, bark, and flowers, sifted and unsifted, powders, capsules, pills, tinctures, tonics, extracts, and more. Dietary supplements may be "natural," but they're still chemicals, and will affect the body in the same manner that synthetic drugs will.

One thing you should know about herbs: Supplement makers are not subject to FDA good manufacturing practices (GMP), as are makers of foods and over-the-counter and prescription drugs. Drugs are standardized; the active ingredient is known, each dose contains the same amount of that ingredient, and each dose has the exact same makeup. Plants are very complicated chemically. If the active ingredient hasn't been identified, as is the case with most herbals, the manufacturer can't provide a standardized product. Further, there is no legal definition of standardization for botanicals.

Botanicals contain hundreds, even thousands, of compounds in varying ratios, depending on where and when they are harvested. The amount of active ingredient varies widely, despite label claims. Quality and content vary from manufacturer to manufacturer, batch to batch. Unlike drugs, most supplement labels don't have consumer warnings describing possible side effects. Some supplements from Asia, perhaps even those you might consider taking for your food allergy symptoms, have been found contaminated with poisonous metals—lead, arsenic, mercury, and drugs unlisted on the label have also been found.

Buyer, Beware

Using herbs to treat allergic symptoms has been in practice for centuries. However, if you are thinking of taking herbs for your food allergies, we can't caution enough: As herbs contain active substances that can trigger side effects and interact with other herbs, supplements, and medications, they must be carefully administered. Especially if you are currently being treated with any medications, you should not use herbal preparations without first discussing the matter with your physician.

Herbal Products and Their Adverse Effects

The following table provides an overview of reported adverse effects of some common herbal products (courtesy of Kaiser Permanente).

continues

continued

Herb	Adverse Effect
Chinese herbs containing Aristolochic acid	Renal failure and cancer
Chinese herbs containing Stephania & Magnolia	Severe kidney injury
Chaparral	Hepatitis
Comfrey	Hepatic veno-occlusive disease and cirrhosis
Ginger, ginseng, feverfew, devil's claw, dong quai	Causes increased bleeding in patients taking aspirin, warfarin, or NSAIDs
St. John's wort	Reduces efficacy of cyclosporine, birth control pills, and protase inhibitors; many other potential drug interactions
Licorice	Hypokalmemia and hypertension
Ephedra	Hypertension
Evening primrose	Seizure
Aconia	Heart failure
Yohimbe	Renal failure, seizures, death; MAO-I could interact with medications and tyramine-containing foods
L-5 hydroytryplotophan	Eosinophilia-mylangia syndrome (EMS)

A Plethora of Plants

Many different herbs have been cited, both in recognized medical literature such as the *Physicians' Desk Reference for Herbs*, as well as the many popular books on the market on herbs, as being effective remedies for symptoms of food allergies. By and large, finding the right herb that works for you is often a trial-and-error endeavor.

The following herbs are touted as being effective for food allergy relief. You may wish to consider them if their profile fits your needs, and if your doctor approves.

- ◆ **Dandelion.** Although many people think the dandelion is just a nuisance weed clogging their lawns, this herb is actually a rich source of vitamins A, B complex, C, and D, as well as minerals such as iron, potassium, and zinc. Native Americans used dandelion to treat swelling, skin problems, heartburn, and gastrointestinal conditions such as stomach upset, flatulence, and constipation; Chinese herbologists likewise use dandelion in treating digestive disorders, and in Europe, dandelion is used for bowel problems.

Dandelion is a natural diuretic that is also a source of potassium, a nutrient often lost with other diuretics. The root of the dandelion plant has laxative effects and is also used to improve digestion. Dandelion herbs are available fresh or dried in a variety of forms, including tinctures, prepared tea, and capsules.

Dandelion is generally considered safe. Some individuals, however, may develop an allergic reaction from touching the herb, and others may develop mouth sores. People with gall bladder conditions such as gallstones should definitely consult their physician before ingesting dandelion.

◆ **Primrose.** Evening primrose has served for centuries in treating upset stomach and respiratory conditions. Today, evening primrose seed oil (EPO) is used to relieve the itch of skin problems like eczema and hives that are frequently caused by a food allergy. It is also used in the treatment of inflammatory bowel disease like ulcerative colitis, which can be another food allergy symptom. Evening primrose oil is extracted from seeds and prepared as medicine using a chemical called hexane and is available as oil or in capsules.

◆ **Flaxseed.** This herb is claimed to be useful for several symptoms of food allergies. Flaxseed is derived from the flax plant. Ancient Egyptians used it for nutritional and laxative purposes. It is high in fiber and a gummy material called mucilage, substances which expand when coming in contact with water, thus adding bulk to stool and helping it move quickly through the gastrointestinal tract. Flaxseed and flaxseed oil is claimed to help reduce inflammation and has been used for asthma, the theory being that it helps to decrease inflammation and improve lung function, which in some cases may be caused by a food allergy.

> **CAUTION**
>
> **Skulls and Bones**
>
> If you're pregnant, breastfeeding, over 60, under 18, and/or taking prescription or OTC drugs, you should seek your doctor's advice before taking any herbs. If you have an autoimmune deficiency, be careful. If you're taking NSAIDs, which thin the blood, herbs such as garlic and ginger, even vitamins like vitamin E, will increase your risk of bleeding.

◆ **Chamomile.** It used to be people would walk a mile for a Camel, or so boasted the ads. Not so today, in this health-conscious society of ours. The well-recognized herb chamomile (both Roman and German chamomile) belongs to the Asteraceae family, which also includes ragweed, echinacea, and feverfew. Chamomile has been used traditionally to treat digestive disorders brought on by a food allergy, as well as skin conditions, including eczema, which can be food allergy-initiated. The herb is available as dried flower heads, tea, liquid extract, or topical ointment, and can be used as an inhalant or paste. A small number of people have allergy to chamomile, so if you are one of these, of course you would not try this herb.

Pep Talk on Peppermint

Peppermint serves as a calming agent to soothe an upset stomach or to aid in digestion. Because it has a numbing effect, it has been used to treat skin irritations, nausea, diarrhea, and flatulence—all of these, of course, being common symptoms of food allergies.

> **Skulls and Bones**
>
> Peppermint tea is usually a safe way to soothe an upset stomach. However, if your symptoms of indigestion are related to gastroesophageal reflux disease (GERD), you shouldn't use peppermint, because it can relax the sphincter muscles between the stomach and esophagus, allowing stomach acids to flow back into the esophagus.

> **Timely Tip**
>
> Some herbs with claims in the form of anecdotal evidence for treating asthma are: bayberry, bloodroot, cayenne, chickweed, colt's foot, comfrey, ephedrine (ephedra), eucalyptus, garlic, ginkgo, gumplant, lobelia, peppermint, Roman chamomile, goldenseal, mullein, sage, saw palmetto, thyme, tobacco, uncaria tomentosa (cat's claw), wild cherry bark, and zizyphus spinosa (jujube).

A few of the many claims of the herb peppermint include the following:

- **For indigestion.** Peppermint calms the muscles of the stomach and improves the flow of bile, aiding the body in digesting fats and enabling food to pass through the stomach more quickly.

- **For flatulence and bloating.** Peppermint relaxes the muscles that allow the body to rid itself of painful digestive gas.

- **For irritable bowel syndrome (IBS).** Studies have shown the beneficial effects of enteric-coated peppermint capsules for treating IBS symptoms, such as pain, bloating, gas, and diarrhea.

- **As a decongestant and expectorant.** Peppermint and its main active agent, menthol, are effective for these purposes.

- **For itching and skin irritations.** When applied topically, peppermint has a soothing effect on hives. Apply menthol, the active ingredient in peppermint, in a cream or ointment. (Menthol or peppermint oil applied directly to the skin can cause contact dermatitis or other type of rash. Also, pure menthol is poisonous and should never be taken internally.)

In summary, if you're going to take herbs:

- Take them on good information.

- Read labels.

- Buy from a reputable manufacturer.

- Keep your doctor informed; report adverse side effects.

- Stay on your regular medications.

Vitamins to the Rescue

Vitamins and supplements have been with us for a long time. Mom and Dad always told us they were good for us, so back then, when we were kids, we resisted taking them. Not any longer. Today, everyone wants to do the utmost to benefit their health, so vitamins play an important role in our health-conscious twenty-first-century society. And the good news is, there are a number of vitamins, minerals, and supplements that can, in one way or another, provide help with your allergy in the form of support. These include acidophilus, omega-3 and omega-6, selenium, folic acid, vitamin C, zinc, and others.

Here is a short breakdown of those vitamins with favorable reports for treating symptoms of a food allergy:

- **Acidophilus.** The breakdown of food by acidophilus leads to production of lactic acid, hydrogen peroxide, and other byproducts that make an environment hostile for undesired organisms. Acidophilus also produces lactase, the enzyme that breaks down milk sugar (lactose) into simple sugars. As individuals who are lactose intolerant don't produce this enzyme, acidophilus supplements may be useful for them. Acidophilus has been used to prevent and treat diarrhea, irritable bowel syndrome, Crohn's disease, and ulcerative colitis, all of which may be caused by or aggravated by a food allergy or intolerance. It is also used for respiratory conditions in lowering the risk of allergies (asthma, hay fever), food allergies to milk, and skin conditions such as eczema.

- **Omega-3/omega-6.** These are essential fatty acids, meaning they are essential to human health but cannot be manufactured by the body, so must be obtained from food. Omega-3 fatty acids are found in fish and certain plant oils. Extensive research indicates that omega-3 fatty acids reduce inflammation in food allergy-induced asthma, and may be helpful in treatment of skin disorders, inflammatory bowel disease, Crohn's disease, and ulcerative colitis, also symptoms of a food allergy. Omega-6 fatty acids may be useful in treating eczema and other food allergies. Consult your doctor for details on dosage.

♦ **Selenium.** Selenium is an essential mineral found in trace amounts in the human body. It works as an antioxidant by scavenging damaging particles in the body known as free radicals and neutralizing them. The body needs selenium for the proper functioning of the immune system and for the production of prostaglandins. Many of the benefits of selenium are related to its role in the production of the enzyme glutathione peroxidase, which is responsible for detoxification in the body. Selenium enhances the immune system's ability to fight illness and infection. It is believed effective in treatment of asthma, inflammatory bowel disease, and skin conditions such as eczema, all related to food allergy/intolerance.

♦ **Folic acid.** Folic acid is also known as vitamin B_9. All the B vitamins help the body to convert carbohydrates into glucose (sugar), which is then used to produce energy. These B vitamins are essential in the breakdown of fats and protein. B complex vitamins also play an important role in maintaining muscle tone along the lining of the digestive tract and promoting the health of the nervous system, skin, eyes, and mouth. Folic acid deficiency is the most common B vitamin deficiency, and can cause the reaction of diarrhea. Irritable bowel syndrome and celiac disease can cause a deficiency of this nutrient.

♦ **Vitamin C.** Vitamin C is needed for the growth and repair of body tissues and forming collagen, an important protein. Vitamin C is an antioxidant, and may be useful boosting immune system functions and treating food allergy-related conditions such as asthma, eczema, and hay fever.

Timely Tip

Look for vitamins and supplements in spray form. Many vitamin pills and capsules don't dissolve in the digestive tract quickly enough to be absorbed, so that by the time the digestive process is completed, only a small percentage of the nutrient actually enters the bloodstream.

♦ **Zinc.** Zinc is an essential trace mineral that must be obtained from diet, since the body can't make enough. Zinc plays an important role in the immune system, and is helpful in protecting against infections. Zinc also has some antioxidant properties, which means that it helps protect cells in the body from the potential damage caused by free radicals. Zinc deficiency can be caused by allergies that interfere with the absorption of nutrients from food, or by conditions such as irritable bowel disease, celiac disease, and chronic diarrhea.

Some other vitamins, minerals, and supplements that are claimed to be helpful to symptoms of food allergy include bromelain, quercetin, thiamine, cobalamin, vitamin B_2, pantothenic acid, pyridoxine, niacinamide, coenzyme Q10, niacin, potassium, vitamin E, and pancretin. These are said to help relieve symptoms of pain, swelling, nausea, and inflammation, and to boost and give support to the immune system.

Sniff a Whiff

Food allergy as well as any chronic medical problem will be made worse by stress. Also, any chronic problem will cause or increase stress levels. This being the case, look for safe ways to relieve the stress level. Here is one approach.

Doctors are unlikely to prescribe aromatherapy, but don't let that stand in the way of using this therapy yourself. You may be pleasantly surprised, for aromatherapy and the products it uses, essential oils, could benefit you in alleviating stress, promoting relaxation, and relieving anxiety and insomnia, which could be byproducts of your food allergy/intolerance. A possible added bonus: Some people have claimed aromatherapy to be an excellent pain reliever.

Aromatherapy treatments use concentrated essential oils extracted from herbs and oils produced using a plant's flowers, leaves, roots, bark, or branches, either by steam distillation or cold pressing. The volatile, flammable oils are mixed with a carrier oil or diluted in alcohol before being used in therapy. You can buy these oils in health food stores, as well as in bulk form from wholesale suppliers, via the Internet, or from ads.

Skulls and Bones
Sage, rosemary, and juniper oils can cause uterine contractions when taken in excessive amounts.

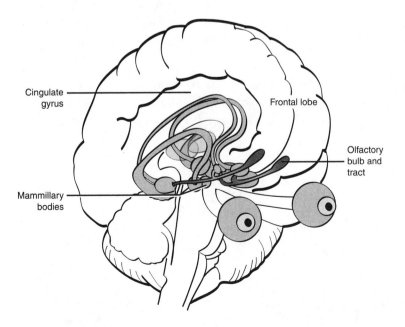

Cingulate gyrus

Frontal lobe

Olfactory bulb and tract

Mammillary bodies

Flared like a wishbone, the limbic system wraps around the top of the brainstem. As emotion is controlled here, many believe that aromatherapy acts on the limbic brain.

Aromatherapy and Its Uses

Some of the different ways to use aromatherapy are:

◆ **Inhalation.** Add a few drops of essential oil to a bowl of steaming water, then place a towel over your head, and breathe in the fragrant vapors.

◆ **Diffusion.** Spray the compounds into the air. Add 10 drops of an essence to 7 tablespoons water, shake the mixture, fill a spray bottle with it, and squirt it around the house.

◆ **Massage.** Most aromatherapy massage preparations contain five drops of essential oil blended with a light oil base. Rubbing this into the skin may be either calming or stimulating, depending on the oil used.

◆ **Bathing.** Add a few drops to your bath, Jacuzzi, hot tub, or foot bath.

◆ **Hot and cold compresses.** Add a few drops of oil to water. Soak a cloth in the solution, then apply to a troubled area.

CAUTION

Skulls and Bones

Do not take aromatherapy oils internally. They are too potent for this kind of use, and some of them could also be poisonous.

While aromatic oils have been used therapeutically for thousands of years, contemporary aromatherapy originated in the 1930s in France and came to the United States in the 1980s. Proponents say aromatherapy heals, stimulates the immune system, relieves pain, reduces swelling, and improves circulation. Its enthusiasts explain that fragrances stimulate the brain via the limbic system, the part of the brain that is the seat of emotion.

Other aromatherapy aficionados suggest that aromas may work by stimulating the adrenals to produce steroidlike hormones that fight pain and inflammation. Others believe that the essential oils react with hormones and enzymes in the bloodstream to alleviate pain.

Each essence is said to accomplish a unique function. Here are some of the common essential oils and their supposed effects, which can be used for the relief of allergy symptoms:

◆ **Lavender.** Relieves inflammation and nausea.

◆ **Peppermint.** Relieves pain.

◆ **Eucalyptus.** Clears sinuses.

◆ **Rosemary.** Relieves pain, lessens swelling.

- **Chamomile.** Reduces swelling, treats allergic symptoms.

- **Everlasting.** Reduces swelling, treats pain.

Oil's Well That Ends Well

Essential oils soothe. Try some lavender oil or peppermint oil. A drop or two is all you need, applied directly to the temples. If you massage using slight pressure in a clockwise direction, you should find relief across the forehead and bridge of the brow.

Proponents of this therapy say that toxins accumulate at the gap between the base of the skull and neck (the occipital ridge), thus massaging provides relief by dislodging the toxins, which are creating tension and pressure felt in the head. A sprinkling of a few drops of lavender's essential oil into a basin of steaming water, then inhaling the vapors, is also said to help clear the head and smells good.

You should be sure to drink plenty of water to help flush the toxins out of your body once they have been dislodged. For an aromatic bath, try lavender oil mixed with rosemary oil and/or peppermint oil. Remember to inhale the vapors deeply, and if it is your bedtime, apply the formula to encourage a restful sleep.

Timely Tip

Bromelain is an enzyme from pineapple that is used as a supplement for reducing inflammation and improving absorption of nutrients. It has been suggested that the speed at which inflammation occurs and is resolved is regulated in the body by hormone-like chemicals called prostaglandins. The body has both good and bad prostaglandins. Bad prostaglandins stimulate pain receptors and encourage inflammation; good prostaglandins inhibit inflammation. It is suggested that bromelain inhibits only the bad prostaglandins and keeps blood platelets from aggregating.

A Few Caveats

You should be aware of the following caveats if you are using essential oils:

- Many essential oils can trigger bronchial spasms. If you have asthma, don't try aromatherapy without consulting your doctor.

- If you have skin allergies, don't use essential oils in your bath.

- Avoid aromatherapy during pregnancy.

- Be careful of using oils on young children, especially on their faces.

- Do not use peppermint oil on children under three; their skin is too delicate to tolerate it.

- Because essential oils are highly concentrated, taking them internally can easily lead to a toxic overdose. Do not ingest even the tiniest amount without your doctor's approval.

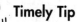

Timely Tip

To check whether you're allergic to an oil or not, place one drop on the inside of your elbow and wait 24 hours to see if it produces a reaction.

- Except for lavender, do not use any highly concentrated, undiluted oils on your skin; they are too potent. Always dilute.

- Keep oils away from your eyes; close your eyes while inhaling aromatic vapors.

- Some essential oils may cause skin irritation if used too frequently. They can also increase your sensitivity to sunlight, making it easier to burn.

The Least You Need to Know

- Herbs, vitamins, and essential oils/aromatherapy are alternative remedies that may help soothe allergy symptoms.

- Much anecdotal evidence exists for the efficacy of the remedies named in this chapter.

- While scientific proofs are lacking, proponents believe these methods have merit.

- Some of these methods can't hurt you; others might. Caution is suggested in some cases; full steam ahead in others.

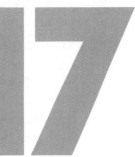
Cornucopia Exotica

In This Chapter

- ◆ Learn how Chinese herbs may be effective for food allergy and food intolerance symptoms
- ◆ Discover the pluses and minuses of India's Ayurvedic medicine
- ◆ Examine homeopathy and its many remedies
- ◆ Decide whether exotic remedies will be helpful to your condition

Chinese herbs, the treatments of Ayurvedic medicine, and homeopathic remedies are so numerous as to require a lifetime of study even to catalog, let alone fully understand. For this reason, we've grouped these exotic remedies into a category that we call *Cornucopia Exotica* and have given it its own chapter.

Many people gravitate to these remedies precisely because they are "different"—purportedly kinder and gentler, and certainly with a greater mystique than the staple but sometimes boring plain old vanilla vitamin. Who wouldn't rather boast to their friends, "I'm taking tienchi ginseng, schizandra berries, wild yam root, magnolia bark, and poria mushroom for my food allergy," than "I'm using vitamin C"?

This chapter provides a closer look at these originally foreign remedies that enjoy so much cachet they are appealing to an ever-widening audience in America. Once again, we must caution that in this chapter, we are not providing any medical advice, and do not advocate the use of any of these treatments without the concurrence of your physician. This chapter is written for information only. If you have a food allergy, you should be treated by a board-certified allergist.

Chinese Herbs to the Rescue

Chinese herbal medicine is traditionally used either as a stand-alone treatment or to implement other modalities, such as acupuncture. Chinese herbal practitioners use different types of information, such as the voice, the pulse, appearance of the tongue, body odors, and the temperature of parts of the body, to tell which herbs are needed. Chinese herbs are determined by a person's whole picture, not just symptoms and signs of illness. Age, sex, constitution, diet, lifestyle, and emotional state all affect which herbs are selected as suited to a problem. Food allergies, a frequently seen complaint in Chinese medicine, are classified either as the invasion of external evils or because of internal disruption.

The six external evils or excesses are wind, cold, summer heat, dampness, dryness, and fire. Internal causes can be due to a disruption of any of the fourteen meridians, because many of the meridians ascend to the head.

Timely Tip

Exotic herbal remedies that can be used for symptoms of a food allergy or food intolerance proliferate, and there is a great deal of anecdotal evidence for them. It's wise to keep in mind that herbology is a lifelong study in itself. Many people take herbal recommendations from the salesperson at their local health food store, but you would do well to bone up and do your own research.

How Safe Is Safe?

Chinese herbal formulas are thousands of years old and are said to have been tested for safety and effectiveness. However, going to a health food store and selecting herbs on your own, if you're not an expert at Chinese herbology, could create problems, because some herbs can be toxic. Furthermore, if you're self-prescribing, your knowledge should include herbal and drug interactions as well. In the field of Chinese herbs, several patent or prepared medicines on the market treat allergies. A word of caution: Many of the formulas contain metal, such as arsenic or lead. Further research is needed to investigate the soil the herbs are grown in, and some products have been banned.

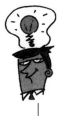

Bet You Didn't Know

The Food and Drug Administration publishes bulletins with results of animal testing and reported adverse reactions in people, attributed and proven. In addition, county health departments and a reporting source that most physicians subscribe to publish new information about all drugs and OTC drugs, herbs, and so on. Based on this, the FDA can ban sale of any drug thought to be harmful.

Esoterica for Allergy

Some of the herbs and herbal combinations mentioned here are likely to be new to you. They aren't as well known as the herbs you've been seeing around for years, but some are coming on strong and are claimed to be effective for food allergy treatment. Here is a list of some of the many Chinese herbal formulas that are used for food allergies:

♦ For regulating stagnant Qi (energy): poria cocos, bupleurem root, atractylodes, chaste berries, dong quai, peony root, cyperus rhizome, black haw bark, wild yam, magnolia bark, ginger, licorice root, green bitter orange peel, ligusticum wallichii, mint leaves, gastrodia. This remedy is often used to treat digestive upset, abdominal distention, belching, gas, nausea, and constipation.

♦ For Qi deficiency: astragalus, ginseng, atractylodes, tangkuei, cimicifuga, bupleurum.

♦ To strengthen the Qi and aid digestion: four nobles or si junza tang, ginseng, codonopsis, atractylodes, poria, licorice.

♦ To tone the Qi, especially of the stomach and immune system: panax ginseng, American ginseng, Siberian ginseng, tienchi ginseng, codonopsis, astragalus, atractylodes, poria mushroom, fo-ti, dong quai, licorice.

♦ To tone the immune system and help produce antibodies: echinacea angustifolia, echinacea palida, echinacea purpurea.

♦ To tone yin and yang, protect the immune system, and aid in antibody production: pau d'arco, echinacea root, astragalus, suma, Siberian ginseng, reishi mushroom, schizandra berries, ligustrum fruit, chaparral, goldenseal, garlic.

♦ To soothe inflammatory conditions, cleanse and tone the immune system, and help produce antibody protection: echinacea angustifolia, echinacea palida, echinacea purpurea.

♦ For cough and asthma (if you have nasal congestion or cough with profuse phlegm, eliminate cinnamon from the formula): ma huang decoction, ma huang, cinnamon branch, apricot seed, licorice.

◆ For respiratory allergies, such as asthma: ma huang, platycodon, comfrey root, mullein, wild cherry bark, licorice, elecampane, ginger, cinnamon twigs, wild ginger root.

◆ A decongestant formula for allergies, especially asthma and upper respiratory problems: ma huang, platycodon, comfrey root, mullein, wild cherry bark, licorice, elecampane, ginger, cinnamon twigs, wild ginger root.

◆ For skin disorders such as eczema (for a weaker individual who has profuse perspiration and coldness): cinnamon branch, peony root, licorice, jujube dates, fresh ginger.

◆ For bloating and diarrhea: ginger root, cinnamon twigs, cayenne, cloves, bayberry bark, white pine bark, marshmallow root, licorice root.

◆ For digestive problems, nausea, vomiting, diarrhea, constipation, bloating and cramps: poria cocos mushroom, coix seed, kudzu, actractylodes, wild yam root, cumin seed, costus root, cardamon seed, magnolia bark, rice sprouts, peppermint leaf, ume plum, gastrodia elata, citrus peel (tangerine or orange).

◆ For congestion, bloating, diarrhea: ginger root, cinnamon twigs, cayenne, cloves, bayberry bark, white pine bark, marshmallow root, licorice root.

◆ To neutralize stomach acids and promote detoxification: dandelion root, violet leaves, black pepper, cleavers, fennel seed, cardamom seed.

Body Movements

If you're all bound up with constipation, it may be due to food allergy or food intolerance. Laxatives such as the following formulas may also help bloating, stomach acid, and other symptoms of food allergy/intolerance. Here are two suggested laxative formulas to help if you're all bound up:

◆ To lubricate dryness and promote bowel elimination: psyllium, flax, chia seeds. Soak three to four tablespoons overnight in a cup of black cherry juice and drink the next day.

◆ For symptoms of a food allergy and intolerance, such as upset stomach, diarrhea, skin eruptions, and many others: rhubarb root, ginger root, licorice root. Cascara sagrada may be substituted for rhubarb if digestive symptoms are present.

Balance with Ayurveda, Ancient Medicine of India

The Ayurvedic medical system aims not merely to treat disease, but to balance the energy and health of mind and body. Derived from ancient theories that originated on the Indian subcontinent, Ayurvedic medicine's goal is prevention of disease through the correct balance of three "irreducible principles" at work in the body, called doshas.

A program of treatments, called panchakarma, stresses purification and rejuvenation. Diet, massage, herbs, meditation, breathing, and intestinal cleansing with laxatives, purgatives, or enemas, are claimed to help detoxify the body.

Ayurvedic practitioners will take your medical history, examine your tongue, and take your pulse. As in Chinese medicine, in Ayurvedic medicine the pulse is a critical diagnostic tool, revealing imbalances in the three basic principles or doshas at work in the body.

Methods used to soothe your food allergy and food intolerance symptoms suggested by an Ayurvedic practitioner might include massage with warm sesame oil; avoidance of the specific foods to which you are allergic, emphasis on others as determined by the practitioner; breathing exercises; and herbal saunas or enemas.

Skulls and Bones _____

Don't jump in head first when an Ayurvedic practitioner recommends purgative treatments. Overuse of laxatives and enemas can lead to serious chemical imbalance within the body. Consult your primary care physician first.

Med Meaning _____

Ayurveda refers to an Indian medical system, meaning knowledge of life. It was first popularized in the United States by the Maharishi Mahesh Yogi, founder of the Transcendental Meditation movement. Later, physician and best-selling author Deepak Chopra began promoting the system in his books and seminars, as well as on television and at his clinics.

Greet Your Doshas

An Ayurvedic practitioner will identify your "tridosha," or unique combination of the three doshas, and prescribe dietary recommendations, exercises, and other therapies designed to bring your tridosha into balance.

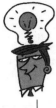

Bet You Didn't Know

According to Ayurveda, there are three doshas, or basic metabolic types: kapha, pitta, and vata. Each dosha is rooted in specific organs of the body. Combinations of these doshas in various proportions comprise a total of 10 body types, which determine each individual's physical and emotional makeup. Remedies are prescribed according to type.

Your tridosha profile will determine your optimum program. Ayurvedic diets are based on foods' flavor, not their nutritional content. Herbal prescriptions are selected from traditional Indian remedies. Purifying the body through excretion is stressed, including herbal enemas and steam treatments. Induced vomiting, a purgative technique used in Indian Ayurvedic practice, is not too popular with American subjects.

The Big Three

Ayurveda's most prevalent and well-known herbs are as follows:

- **Triphala.** This translates as "three fruits" and consists of the combination of the fruit of the chebulic, beleric, and emblic myrobalan trees, known in India as harad, behada, and amla, respectively. Triphala is used as a laxative. It is a formula for cleansing, detoxifying, and promoting digestion.

- **Chyavanprash.** To tone spleen and stomach Qi. Chyavanprash is made with fresh Indian gooseberries called amla or amlakis. These fruits are considered the major health food herb throughout India and are the highest known source of easily digested vitamin C. Hundreds of fresh amla fruits are cleaned, washed, and tied in a cloth, boiled in water slowly until reduced to one-sixth the original volume. The substance is then strained, and seeds removed and discarded. The fruit is fried in sesame oil and butter and reduced to a paste. This paste, combined with the remaining decoction, is further boiled and reduced with jaggury (crude brown sugar with molasses). Approximately 34 to 50 herbs, depending on which variant of Chyavanprash is used, are added in powder form. The preparation is well cooked and honey is added to complete the process of manufacture.

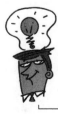

Bet You Didn't Know

In India and China, health-care professionals use modern Western medical techniques along with their own traditional ones.

Ancient Sanskrit texts prescribe Chyavanprash's regular use for allergies and immune weakness. It affects regularity of bowel movements, removes parasites and toxins, and cures indigestion and dyspepsia.

◆ **Guggula.** Guggula is made from the resin of Balsaodendron Mukul, and is closely related to myrrh. It helps alleviate accumulated cholesterol, thickened mucus, and other materials. Combined with triphala, it is used to counteract constipation.

Cleanse with Ayurveda

No getting around it, Ayurvedic practitioners are strong believers in cleansing of every body orifice possible. Practitioners consider enema therapy a complete treatment for many symptoms, including constipation and distention.

There are three basic types of Ayurvedic enemas:

◆ **Oil enema.** A cup of warm sesame or other oil is used.

◆ **Decoction enema.** An herb tea, taken rectally.

◆ **Nutritive enema.** Mix warm milk with meat broth or bone marrow soup.

If enemas are not your cup of tea, here are a few nonenema Ayurvedic formulas:

◆ To relieve gas, bloating, and indigestion, to remove mucus, and to treat allergies: ginger root, black pepper, pippli long pepper, honey.

◆ For food allergy relief: asafoedita, atractylodes, cumin seed, caraway seed, pippli long pepper, black pepper, ginger root, dandelion root, slippery elm, green citrus peel, rock salt.

◆ To tone and regulate digestive Qi and eliminate gas and bloating: atractylodes, caraway seed, cumin seed, asafoetida, black pepper, citrus peel, dandelion root, slippery elm, rock salt, ginger.

The neem tree has been used for medicinal purposes for centuries; anecdotal reports date back to the Middle Ages. On the Indian subcontinent, where the neem tree is known as the "village pharmacy," researchers have found more than sixty medicinal uses for the exotic herb.

Extracts of neem leaves are said to reduce anxiety and stress when ingested in small quantities. This may be due to neem's ability to increase the amount of serotonin in the brain, but neem extracts for antianxiety will only work in small doses.

Timely Tip

Along with your allergy, are you a diabetic? Do you suffer from heart disease? Consult your physician and/or registered dietitian before you launch an Ayurvedic diet plan. Ayurvedic recommendations are based mainly on food flavor, thus they may be at odds with your allergy-based needs.

Inhibition by limonoids (and/or polysaccharides) reduces perceived pain. Neem leaf and bark extracts have been shown to be a more potent inhibitor of pain than acetyl-salicylic acid (aspirin) and pethidine hydrochloride. Neem reduces the activity of the central nervous system, which also reduces perceived pain. According to studies in India, neem produces an analgesic effect upon the central and peripheral neural pathways. Indian doctors claim that both opioid and nonopioid receptors can be affected by neem. Widely available in India, neem products until recently were virtually absent from the American market.

Home Sweet Homeopathy

Homeopathy was formulated 200 years ago by German physician Samuel Hahnemann.

Homeopathy arrived in the United States in 1825 through doctors returning from study abroad. Schools were established here; a medical organization was formed. By the mid-1800s, quite a number of U.S. medical schools taught homeopathy. By 1900, the United States had 22 homeopathic medical colleges, and 1 out of 5 doctors were using homeopathy in their practices.

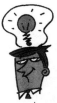

Bet You Didn't Know

To this day, homeopathy remains so popular in Germany that it's impossible to visit even the smallest village that doesn't have at least one or more home-opathic pharmacies conveniently located in the center of town.

Unlike vitamins and herbal remedies, which are sold as dietary supplements, homeopathic remedies are purchased as over-the-counter medications with a unique exemption from standard regulatory procedures. This happened in 1938, through the efforts of U.S. Senator Royal Copeland of New York, a homeopath, who pushed through a special clause in the Federal Food, Drug, and Cosmetic Act that remains in effect today.

Proving and the Law of Infinitesimals

Back in 1800, Dr. Hahnemann noted that a malaria remedy produced malarialike symptoms when taken by a healthy volunteer, which led to the doctor's famous conclusion that "like cures like." Dr. Hahnemann tested substances on himself and others, which bore out his theory of "proving."

Hahnemann's experiments led to his "Law of Infinitesimals," and to the conclusion that the more diluted a substance is, the more powerful its healing action will be. The therapeutic action of homeopathic remedies are attributed to an essence or energy imprint that can mobilize the body's vital forces.

Homeopathy is based on the Law of Similars. Samuel Hahnemann described this principle by using a Latin phrase: *Similia similibus curentur,* which translates as "Let likes cure likes." An example in conventional medicine of "like curing like" is vaccination, and again in conventional medicine, smaller doses of some drugs (such as aspirin to prevent heart attack) are more effective than larger doses or at least safer to the lining of the GI tract. Originally allergy injections were theorized to work on this principle. Subsequently this has proven not to be the way they work. Actually, in allergy shots, the higher the dose the better the success.

Trace Memory Triumphs

Homeopathic medicines are concocted by homeopathic pharmacies in accordance with the processes described in the Homeopathic Pharmacopoeia of the United States, the official manufacturing manual recognized by the FDA.

Substances may be made from plants, minerals, animals (including the venom of poisonous snakes), or chemicals. These substances are highly diluted in a process called *succussion,* so that little of the original remains; however, the solutions continue to hold a trace memory or essence of the original substance.

Med Meaning _____

An original substance, mixed in alcohol, yields a tincture. One drop mixed with 99 drops of alcohol achieves a ratio of 1:100. The mixture is shaken in a process known as **succussion.** The process is repeated numerous times, until a dilution of at least 1 part in 1 million is reached, or even 1 part in 1 trillion. After the succussion process, small sugar globules are saturated with the multi-diluted liquid. This is your homeopathic remedy.

Hundreds of Choices, Which to Choose?

For food allergies, a hundred or more different homeopathic approaches are available, depending on the findings your individual practitioner uncovers.

A homeopathic remedy for a food allergy often includes such esoteric sounding, mostly Latin names as alumina; indigo; cocaine (really!); aconitum napellus; argentum nitricum; platinum metallicum; lycopodium clavatum; adrenalium, arsenicum album, lycopodicum; pusstilla; histamium—and to expose you to antigens: butter, cheese, cow's milk, egg white, egg yolk, yogurt, and/or whatever other substances to which you might be allergic.

Homeopathic How-To

Many homeopathic physicians suggest that remedies be used as follows: Take one dose and wait for a response. If improvement is seen, continue to wait and let the remedy work. If improvement lags significantly or has clearly stopped, another dose may be taken. The frequency of dosage varies with the condition and the individual. Sometimes a dose may be required several times an hour; other times a dose may be indicated several times a day; and in some situations, one dose per day (or less) can be sufficient. If no response is seen within a reasonable amount of time, select a different remedy.

Sensitize Yourself and Make Your Symptoms Go Kaput

Homeopathy seeks to naturally stimulate the body's natural defenses against food allergy symptoms. Homeopathic food allergy remedies are said to place the body in a position to react less to the allergens. Specific homeopathic food allergy remedies include specific allergens to gently, safely expose the individual to their weak areas, thereby allowing the body's natural defenses to properly adapt to the allergen and hopefully no longer react to it adversely.

> **Skulls and Bones**
>
> Few peer review studies exist on the use of Ayurvedic medicines, and many Ayurvedic herbs have potent effects when overused. If you should develop side effects—which may range from drowsiness to nausea—while taking an Ayurvedic remedy, see your allergist at once.

Homeopathy says that digestive problems, inflammation of mucous membranes, itching, and other discomforts due to food allergies occur because of an exaggerated immune response.

For food allergies, a hundred or more different homeopathic approaches are available. The remedies listed in the following section may give you some idea of how homeopathy would attempt to treat food allergy problems.

Homeopathic remedies may be purchased as both singular remedies and combination ones. Following are some single remedies that homeopaths recommend for allergies.

Homeopathic Remedies

The following homeopathic remedies lead the pack:

- ◆ **Allium cepa.** Derived from red onion, it is useful for allergic symptoms of runny nose, excess mucous, and watery eyes, which may result from a food allergy.

◆ **Arsenicum album.** Homeopathy recommends this remedy to people with multiple food allergies, especially when they also feel restless and exhausted. They claim that asthma and digestive disorders (such as vomiting and diarrhea) are common reactions of a food allergy. This remedy is also recommended for eczema and for wheezing due to asthma, both of which are food allergic symptoms.

◆ **Antimonium.** For bronchial mucus discharge from food allergen exposure.

◆ **Arnica.** For inflammation of mucous membranes caused by a food allergy.

◆ **Calcarea carbonica.** This remedy for a food allergy is said to be helpful to people who have become fatigued and overwhelmed. The remedy is especially helpful to those with gastrointestinal symptoms of a food allergy, who are bloated with gas, especially after eating wheat or dairy products to which they are allergic.

◆ **Calcarea phosphorica.** Irritability, headaches, and stomach and abdominal pains are all indications for this remedy. Food allergy symptoms manifesting as gastrointestinal distress are said to be helped with this remedy.

◆ **Carbo vegetabilis.** A person whose food allergy problem involves either digestive or respiratory symptoms may be helped by this remedy. Bloating, flatulence, and a frequent need to burp are common symptoms. Breathing may be difficult. The person may also feel roughness in the larynx, or weakness or burning in the chest due to asthma.

◆ **Gelsium.** Food allergy reactions with flulike symptoms may indicate a need for this remedy, say homeopathy practitioners.

◆ **Hepar sulphuris calcareum.** People who need this remedy can have skin problems or respiratory problems. A yellow discharge and offensive sour or cheeselike odors are often seen as food allergy symptoms that respond to this treatment. The odor is the sulfa.

◆ **Lycopodium.** Food allergy problems with heartburn, gas, and abdominal cramps could indicate a need for this remedy. The patient feels hunger, yet quickly gets bloated from eating a very small amount. This person may also experience a constricted feeling in the chest, and have difficulty with coughing and breathing.

◆ **Lappa.** For skin rashes from food allergies.

◆ **Ledum.** For cough resulting from food allergies.

◆ **Natrum carbonicum.** This remedy can be helpful to people who have indigestion and heartburn when offending foods are eaten. For instance, milk or dairy products result in flatulence or diarrhea.

◆ **Natrum muriaticum.** A person who needs this remedy can react to food allergens with hay fever symptoms or respiratory problems. Asthma attacks due to a food allergy may be worse in the early evening. It is said that a craving for salt and very strong thirst may help to confirm the choice of this remedy.

◆ **Natrum mur.** This remedy is said to be effective for those with chronic food allergy manifesting in respiratory symptoms such as hay fever; for runny nose, watery eyes, and excess mucous. It is recommended for food allergic reactions of sneezing, obstructed nose, itching in eyes, dry larynx, mucous in the larynx, and dry cough, and is also useful in treating constipation resulting from a food allergy.

◆ **Nux moschata.** If a person reacts to food allergen exposure with an overwhelming feeling of sleepiness, this remedy should be considered. A very dry mouth, dry eyes, a feeling of weight in the chest, and numbness in the extremities are other indications. Constipation resulting from a food allergy might be another symptom.

◆ **Nux vomica.** Irritability, cramping pains, and chilliness are typical symptoms that manifest when this remedy is needed. Oversensitivity to food substances can lead to many ailments—runny nose, tight breathing, heartburn, stomach problems, or constipation.

◆ **Petroleum.** A person who needs this may experience the food allergy reactions of diarrhea and nausea. Individuals who need this remedy to help their food allergy problems have often developed eczema with inflamed and cracking skin, especially on the palms and fingertips.

◆ **Phosphorus.** People who need this remedy may have respiratory problems, nausea, or diarrhea caused by a food allergy.

◆ **Silicea** (also called **Silica**). This remedy is claimed to be helpful to individuals with low stamina, who are prone to fatigue, and whose resistance to infection may be poor. A strong craving for sweets also fits the profile of one who needs this remedy.

◆ **Sulphur.** For food allergic reactions in breathing and skin, especially for irregular breathing relief due to asthma.

◆ **Selenium.** For chest discomfort and coughs resulting from a food allergy.

◆ **Sepia.** For those whose nausea improves from vomiting, eating, or exertion.

Bet You Didn't Know

Homeopathy is popular in many European countries, including Great Britain, and it is a well-publicized fact that members of the royal family are firm advocates of homeopathy. Prince Charles, Prince Philip, the Queen, the late Queen Mother, Princess Margaret, and Princess Diana are a few of the royals on record to have sworn by these treatments.

Some additional single remedies that may help food allergy sufferers include the following:

♦ **Thuja.** For asthma.

♦ **Histaminum.** For nasal congestion.

♦ **Graphites.** For skin symptoms, including painful skin cracks due to eczema.

Homeopathic Combos

At your health food counter, you will find such homeopathic combination remedies as these:

♦ **Adrenalinum, Allium cepa, Arsenicum iod, Euphrasia.** For burning, red itchy eyes; for excess mucous, runny nose; for indigestion. Lessens symptoms such as sneezing, itchy eyes, congestion, sinus pressure, and hay fever.

♦ **Allium cepa, Arsenicum iodatum, Euphrasia, Sabadilla.** For relieving symptoms of runny nose, sneezing, itchy and watery eyes, respiratory congestion, and for relief of allergy and hay fever symptoms, such as difficulty breathing; also used for rashes. Can be taken prior to exposure as a preventative measure.

♦ **Euphrasia and Allium.** Helps strengthen resistance to food allergens, at the same time relieving itchy, watery eyes and respiratory congestion.

♦ **Lycopodium, Natrum sulphur, Silicea.** To desensitize the body from food allergy reactions, to relieve symptoms of runny nose, respiratory congestion, itchy eyes, and difficulty breathing.

Getting Nosey

You might also want to try one of these homeopathic nasal sprays:

♦ **Hay fever nasal spray containing homeopathic histaminum.** To clear out excess mucous in the sinuses and throat, for nasal congestion, runny nose, sneezing, watery eyes, and excess mucous in throat and for asthma and other respiratory symptoms of food allergy; galphimia glauca for asthma and hay fever; luffa for rhinitis and nasal inflammations; sulphur for nasal congestion and burning and red eyes.

♦ **Nasal spray for sinus relief.** Euphorbium for relief of nasal passages and to restore free breathing and eliminate congestion. Ingredients include: euphorbium officinarum for itching in the nose, sneezing, runny nose, and to open nasal passages in cases of rhinitis and sinusitis; pulsatilla for sinus pressure, plugged-up ears, cough, runny nose, excess yellow or green mucus; hepar sulph for pain in nose; argentum nit for congestion; mucosa nasalis and sinusitusinum for respiratory support.

Mix Your Own

You may order specific homeopathic potentized allergens for your own particular food sensitivity. It is said that these potentized remedies from specific antigens can help induce an immune response in individuals suffering from food allergies. Homeopathy allows you to choose from hundreds of available allergens. For instance: apple, almond, ash tree, beef, birch tree, brazil nut, butter, cashew nut, cheddar cheese, cola nut, corn, hazelnut, peanut, pecan, pineapple, potato, ragweed mix, raisin, salmon, silk, tomato, tuna, vanilla, vinegar, walnut, wasp, wheat, wheat pollen, red wine, wool, baker's yeast, brewer's yeast, and yogurt, to mention just a few.

The Least You Need to Know

- ◆ Homeopathy is safe and its proponents claim to have had success in treating food allergies.

- ◆ Traditional Chinese medicine may give support to your allergy symptoms.

- ◆ Indian Ayurvedic medicine has been known to relieve allergic symptoms.

- ◆ Always consult your allergist or physician before using any of the aforementioned techniques—some may be inadvisable in your case.

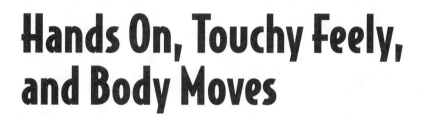

Chapter 18

Hands On, Touchy Feely, and Body Moves

In This Chapter

- ◆ Using traditional Chinese medicine
- ◆ Massaging away pain Japanese and Swedish style
- ◆ Practicing yoga for allergy relief
- ◆ Exploring reflexology and rolfing for allergy relief

Over the past four decades, more and more Americans have experimented with or turned to the Asian traditions of acupuncture, Shiatsu, and yoga in their search for a healthier body and life. Many of these Far Eastern disciplines can be valuable adjuncts to conventional therapy for food allergies, can promote wellness, and help heal symptoms, if administered by qualified practitioners. Thus are the claims of the proponents of these therapies.

The alternative modalities discussed in this chapter share something in common, in that all are considered hands on, touchy feely, and/or body movement techniques, all aim to enhance your feeling of well-being, and all can be considered complementary, because they blend well with treatments for food allergies and food intolerance recommended by orthodox medicine.

Among the food allergy/intolerance symptoms that may find relief using the therapies featured in this chapter are nausea, bloating, gas, and other gastrointestinal as well as respiratory disorders.

However, if you decide to give one or more of these alternatives a try, you should first consult with your physician, especially if you have symptoms of chest pain, shortness of breath, wheezing, constant headache, associated loss of vision or loss of balance, stomach pain with weight loss, or any other abnormal symptoms. In some instances, these complementary disciplines may be not be recommended for you. As with the previous chapters in this part, the content presented here is for your information only. Neither the authors nor the publisher are endorsing or suggesting these forms of therapy.

The Healing Powers of Traditional Chinese Medicine

Traditional Chinese medicine (TCM) began at least 4,000 to 5,000 years ago, when Taoist priests in northern China created QiGong, a form of meditative movement used to cultivate the life force, called *Qi* (pronounced *tchee*). Since then, many other branches of TCM have developed, including acupuncture, acupressure, moxibustion, and tai chi chu'an. All these branches of TCM aim to strengthen the immune system to prevent discomfort, disorder, and disease. It is claimed that all have their use in treating symptoms of food allergies and lessening the distress caused by such symptoms.

Miles of Meridians

According to TCM practitioners, Qi invigorates our bodies through a network of energy channels called meridians. This network spans the entirety of the body, flowing from organ system to organ system, connecting with every cell of the body. TCM is based on the principle that illness is caused by an imbalance of Qi. Stagnant Qi, it is believed, causes malfunction, including food allergies, food intolerance, and other adverse reactions to food.

Med Meaning

Traditional Chinese medicine (TCM) aims to strengthen the immune system to prevent adverse physical, emotional, and spiritual discomfort. **Qi** is the life energy and vital force present within all of nature, including our bodies.

Along the meridians are pressure points or gateways, where Qi can become blocked. With the help of TCM, Qi's flow can be unblocked and balance restored. In this manner, symptoms caused by adverse reactions to food are relieved.

TCM practitioners maintain that by cultivating Qi, we strengthen our body to work better, our immune system gets stronger, our energy level grows, and we have a greater sense of well-being. In this manner, we can discourage allergies from striking. With Chinese medicine, and especially with acupuncture, we can turn our Qi up or down and cause balance to return if we're out of balance.

East Meets West

Proponents of Chinese medicine say that Western medicine is based on the use of chemical and surgical techniques to eliminate disease and promote health, whereas Chinese medicine is less invasive. Chinese medical techniques work slower, it is said, allowing the body to heal itself. By contrast, in Western medicine, prescription drugs take over the task of what the body, if left alone, would be doing for itself. While prescription drugs may have strong side effects and eventually, in some cases, weaken the body, TCM causes none of these disadvantages.

Some Western physicians have been slow to recommend Asian methods of healing. Nevertheless, results experienced by many users verify its effectiveness. This is especially true in the field of chronic pain management.

The diagnostic process used by practitioners of the various branches of TCM may include questioning (medical history, lifestyle), observations (skin, tongue, color), listening (breathing sounds), and pulse-taking. Six pulse aspects said to correlate with body organs or functions are checked on each wrist to determine which meridians are "deficient" in Qi. (Western medicine recognizes only one pulse, corresponding to the heartbeat, which can be felt in the wrist, neck, feet, and various other places.) Some practitioners state that the electrical properties of the body may become imbalanced weeks or even months before symptoms occur.

Sound the Gong for QiGong

Two forms of QiGong, internal and external QiGong, are said to reduce stress and anxiety while improving physical conditions, including those that occur due to adverse food reactions. Internal QiGong involves deep breathing, concentration, and relaxation techniques used by individuals for themselves. External QiGong is performed by "QiGong masters" who claim to cure a wide variety of diseases with energy released from their fingertips.

By alleviating tension, QiGong exercises may relieve pain and other food allergy and food intolerance symptoms, such as indigestion, constipation, diarrhea, nausea, inflammation, and respiratory symptoms.

More than 3,000 techniques exist that can be adapted to the individual. Meditation, visualization, breathing, and movement exercises seek to break down blockages in the flow of Qi and reestablish a healthy supply to distressed parts of the body. (If you're interested in QiGong, check out *The Complete Idiot's Guide to T'ai Chi and QiGong, Second Edition*, by Bill Douglas.)

Proponents say that QiGong heals through enhanced oxygenation of the tissues, and has a beneficial effect on nerves that regulate the pain response. By increasing the flow of lymphatic fluid, QiGong improves the immune system. Helping circulation, it speeds up elimination of toxic substances from the body.

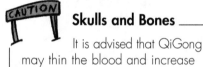

Skulls and Bones

It is advised that QiGong may thin the blood and increase circulation. Do not practice it after a tooth extraction or injury, or when suffering from internal bleeding. Abstain during pregnancy.

Some adherents claim that QiGong moderates the function of the hypothalamus, pituitary, and pineal glands, as well as the fluid surrounding the brain and spinal cord, to decrease pain, increase immunity, and relieve gastrointestinal and respiratory symptoms caused by adverse food reactions of allergy/intolerance.

Acu-Assets

Acupuncture, one of the primary branches of TCM, is a method of inserting sterile needles into points on the body along the meridian channels. This way, Qi is regulated, and discomfort and disorder, including those that may be caused by food allergies, are treated. Along the meridian pathways, close to the surface of the skin, are small nodules called acupressure points that a trained finger can feel. Originally there were 365 such points, corresponding to the days of the year, but the number identified by proponents during the past 2,000 years has increased gradually to around 2,000. Acupuncturists use different types of information, such as the voice, the pulse, appearance of the tongue, odors, and the temperature of parts of the body to diagnose before inserting the needles.

Acupuncture is a choice for many seeking complementary treatments who suffer from food allergy and food intolerance symptoms, including respiratory and gastrointestinal problems. This should not be used to the exclusion of conventional medicine.

Acupuncture can counter pain and swelling. Conditions which are claimed to respond to acupuncture also include gastrointestinal symptoms of food allergies and food intolerance, such as indigestion, constipation, and diarrhea.

The How of Healing

Improperly performed acupuncture can cause fainting, local hematoma due to bleeding from a punctured blood vessel (hematoma is internal bleeding that marks the outer layer of the skin in red patches), pneumo-thorax (punctured lung), convulsions, infections, hepatitis B (from unsterile needles), bacterial endocarditis (infection of a heart valve), contact dermatitis, and nerve damage. These adverse effects are all related to the skills of the acupuncturist.

Bet You Didn't Know

In China, TCM masters have their own medical association, and many hospitals use their services for routine treatment.

Pressing On with Acupressure

Sometimes referred to as "acupuncture without needles," acupressure is claimed to help heal symptoms of food allergies and food intolerance by applying deep finger pressure at "acupoints" located along the fourteen meridians where the body's vital energy or Qi flows, connecting vital organs throughout the body.

Acupressure can be a complement to conventional Western medical treatments for food allergies and food intolerance. Clinical studies of acupressure have brought excellent results in the treatment of nausea and vomiting resulting from adverse food reactions; pressure at a special point on the inside of the wrist has been shown to relieve pain as well. It is claimed that acupressure has also been used for relief of respiratory symptoms caused by food allergy and food intolerance.

Skulls and Bones

Acupressure treatments may involve forceful pressure, thus may not be wise for the elderly or anyone with brittle bones or a spinal injury. Acupressure should also be avoided if you have a bleeding disorder, take anticoagulant drugs, or are undergoing long-term steroid therapy, which can make the bones and tissues fragile.

Shiatsu: Therapeutic Art of Japan

The Japanese healing art of Shiatsu is rooted in TCM. Incorporating therapeutic massage, meditation, and self-healing, Shiatsu aims to clear and balance the patient's vital life force, which in Japan is called *ki*.

In the tenth century, Japanese monks studying Buddhism in China observed the healing methods of TCM and took them back to Japan. The Japanese adopted TCM and enhanced it with new ideas, eventually achieving a unique Japanese form called *Shiatsu*. Combining principles of acupressure, Shiatsu is performed without needles.

Med Meaning

Shiatsu refers to the Japanese art of healing, incorporating therapeutic massage, meditation, and self-healing to clear and balance the life force. In Japanese, *shi* means "hand," and *atsu* means "pressure."

Reiki is Japanese for universal life energy. The Japanese character for *Rei* means universal, transcendental spirit, mysterious power, essence. *Ki* is the vital life energy. It is claimed that this energy increases the body's natural ability to heal physical ailments such as those symptoms caused by food allergy and food intolerance, primarily gastrointestinal and respiratory ones, respectively.

The ancient healing technique of Reiki was rediscovered by Dr. Mikao Usui (1862–1926), who developed the Usui System of Reiki in Japan. After World War II, the Reiki movement was introduced to the West.

Yo! Go, Yoga

An Indian discipline more than 5,000 years old, yoga has penetrated our culture in the last 40 years. Derived from the Sanskrit word for union, yoga is practiced in the United States today primarily for its health benefits, including relief from pain, gastrointestinal and respiratory disorders, and other troublesome possible symptoms of food allergies and food intolerance.

Many symptoms of food allergies and food intolerance cause stress and internal "contraction." Aiming for release of these inner stresses, yoga relieves symptoms by improving tight muscles and circulation, releasing endorphins, and promoting relaxation.

Poses That Heal

If yoga intrigues you, it shouldn't be hard to find classes at your local gym or adult learning center. You may also want to join in one of the cable TV yoga exercise classes or purchase one of the many yoga videotapes on the market. With its proven health benefits, yoga is often used as supplementary therapy for food allergy relief. If you take up yoga for this reason, some of the names of the yoga positions you may do that can help your food allergy symptoms include the following:

♦ **Fish pose.** Relieves upper respiratory congestion and drains the sinuses.

♦ **Headstand.** Allows a supply of oxygen-rich blood to reach your head and brain, and is considered to be a panacea for countless human ills.

♦ **Shoulder stand.** Relieves constipation.

♦ **Thunderbolt pose.** Helps digestive problems and prevents or relieves constipation.

♦ **Seated forward bend.** Improves digestive symptoms.

♦ **Bow position.** Good for respiratory symptoms, lungs, and chest; helps digestion and is good for abdominal distress.

♦ **Wind-release position.** Helps abdominal distress.

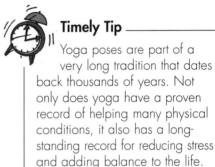

Timely Tip

Yoga poses are part of a very long tradition that dates back thousands of years. Not only does yoga have a proven record of helping many physical conditions, it also has a long-standing record for reducing stress and adding balance to the life.

The Complete Idiot's Guide to Yoga, Third Edition, recommends the following poses for symptoms of allergy, asthma, and respiratory problems: Tree and Warrior poses; Fish, Bow, and Cobra poses. The Lion Pose is said to help throat problems and strengthen the respiratory system, and relieves respiratory distress.

Enter the Endorphins

Yoga produces measurable physiological changes in the body, including a decrease in respiratory rate and blood pressure and an alteration in brain-wave activity reflecting increased relaxation. Yoga is recommended by some yoga practitioners as an adjunct to food allergy therapy. One reason yoga helps may be that it promotes the release of endorphins, the brain's natural painkillers.

Massage Therapy—Rubs You the Right Way

It is claimed that massage provides relief of symptoms caused by adverse food reactions, including associated symptoms of pain and respiratory and gastrointestinal disorders.

Just what is massage? It is the application of pressure to the soft tissues. Through various techniques of kneading, rolling, pounding, pressing, stroking, shaking, drumming, chopping, and striking, healing is promoted through the stimulation of blood and lymph flow to the nerves and tissues, and by loosening muscles. Massage is claimed to enhance the immune system; thus its healing action is claimed to be seen in the relief of many symptoms caused by adverse food reactions. Among these are nausea, bloating, gas, diarrhea, and constipation.

Massage, Swedish Style

The modern principles of Swedish massage include the following:

- **Effleurage.** Slow, rhythmic strokes in the direction of blood flow toward the heart in which the palm and fingers gradually increase pressure.

> **Bet You Didn't Know**
>
> The healing powers of massage have been recognized since antiquity. Massage was used by the ancient Chinese, Egyptians, Greeks, and Romans. In the fifth century B.C.E., Hippocrates, the father of medicine, advised that physicians should be experienced "in rubbing—for rubbing can bind a joint that is too loose, and loosen a joint that is too rigid."

- **Petrissage.** Kneading, pressing, and rolling muscle groups. The grip on the tissues is alternately tightened and loosened.

- **Friction.** A steady pressure or tight circular movements applied across muscle fibers; used in areas near the joints.

- **Tapotement.** Drumming hand movements in which the masseur/masseuse may beat with the fists, strike with fingertips and heel of the hand, and chop or clap.

- **Vibration and jostling.** Vibration entails rapid movements to transmit an oscillating action; mechanical vibrators may also be used. Jostling is rapid shaking of a muscle back and forth.

Swedish massage incorporates long, smooth kneading and stroking hand movements to stimulate lymph circulation. In this technique, manipulation of the soft tissues, combined with active and passive joint movements, improve the functioning of the nervous, muscular, and circulatory systems, which is claimed to help symptoms of food allergies and food intolerance.

Kneading or Not

Circulatory ailments such as phlebitis or varicose veins preclude the use of massage, nor should massage be performed directly over bruises, inflamed or infected injuries, areas of bleeding or heavy tissue damage, or at the site of fractures or sprains. Massage can aggravate existing swelling, and the pressure on the skin can be painful for a person with hives, eczema, or nerve injury. Also avoid massage over tumors and areas of surgical incision.

Abdominal massage should be avoided during the first three months of pregnancy, and possibly during the entire pregnancy, depending on your obstetrician's advice.

Skulls and Bones

If you have a tendency to clotting in the circulatory system, be sure to advise your practitioner, as treatment may be contraindicated.

Reflect on Reflexology

Many health-care practitioners agree that a large percentage of health problems today can be linked to stress and tension. When we fail to manage stress, the body's defense mechanism begins to break down, making us more susceptible to adverse medical conditions. Many people have turned to reflexology as a means of relieving high levels of stress and tension.

Down-Home Homeostasis

Homeostasis is a state of balance. From ancient illustrations and artifacts we know the early Chinese, Japanese, and Egyptians worked on the feet and hands to promote better health. The philosophy of reflexology is often misunderstood as being "foot massage."

Reflexology is based on theories that nerve pathways exist throughout the body. When any of those pathways become blocked, the body experiences discomfort. Reflexology may assist in reviving one's energy flow and bringing the body back into homeostasis, a state of balance.

Feet First

Following are several areas upon which reflexology focuses in their treatments, and the parts of the body to which they correspond:

- **Metatarsal** (balls of the feet). Chest, lung, and shoulder area
- **Toes.** Head and neck
- **Upper arch.** Diaphragm, upper abdominal organs
- **Lower arch.** Pelvic and lower abdominal organs
- **Heel.** Pelvic and sciatic nerve

- **Outer foot.** Arm, shoulder, hip, leg, knee, and lower back

- **Inner foot.** Spine

- **Ankle.** Reproductive organs and pelvic region

Reflexology is both a science and a healing art, based on the theory that there are reflex areas in the feet that correspond to all the glands and organs in the body, and that these areas are responsive to stimulus. Corresponding reflexes are located in the hands.

Timely Tip

Professional reflexologists never diagnose, prescribe, or claim to cure. If you're trying self-reflexology, be aware that some reflexes may be difficult to reach on your own.

The technique improves circulation, increases energy levels, decreases pain, and helps the body achieve balance, so that symptoms of food allergies and food intolerance may be better tolerated. If you suffer from gastrointestinal distress of any sort, including constipation, bloating, gas, diarrhea, or if you have allergic symptoms of a respiratory nature, reflexology may help provide you relief.

The Least You Need to Know

- Several methods of Chinese medicine exist which could help your allergy pain and discomfort.

- Japanese massage is worth trying for certain symptoms.

- Massage therapy, whether in the form of Swedish, neuromuscular, deep tissue, or other system, can be helpful to dealing with your allergies.

- Yoga is beneficial to the body and is effective in complementing allergy treatment.

- Reflexology, and other similar systems, may be effective adjuncts for your allergy condition.

19

Over the Borderline

In This Chapter

- ◆ Explore more complementary therapies
- ◆ Learn about colon cleansing and coffee enemas
- ◆ Decide whether chelation and cell therapy can help your food allergy
- ◆ Find out whether hydrotherapy, hydrothermia, and hypnotherapy could help your food allergy

The therapies featured in this chapter might be classified as "borderline" or "thinking makes it so." It must be emphasized that none of these modalities are recognized by mainstream medicine as effective treatments for symptoms of food allergy, despite the fact that all claim strong adherents. Some of these therapies can't harm, whereas under some circumstances, others could be contraindicated, especially if you should seek such treatments in place of medical solutions. Some of the profiled therapies might make you feel better—soothed and more relaxed. However, none has been scientifically proven to do all they claim they do, although anecdotal evidence in the form of consumer satisfaction is available for all. In other words, it's up to you—and your doctor—whether you want to explore these alternatives. To paraphrase, "we report; you decide."

You probably know that symptomatic relief often depends on mental and psychological outlook. Therefore, belief in an alternative or complementary treatment can be the decisive factor that makes a modality "work" for the believer, as much as faith healing does. Often our minds need a "focal point" to stimulate the healing process. Just remember, food allergy is an immune response, so technically speaking, it cannot be "cured." But if your conviction as to the efficacy of treatments presented in this chapter is strong enough, who knows … the placebo effect might take hold, and you could, miraculously, end up feeling better with your food allergy symptoms relieved. Just keep in mind, however, that none of the modalities in this chapter are in any way substitutes for medical treatment, and the guidance of a qualified allergist is always first and foremost recommended.

Flush That Toosh

Enemas. Surely you've heard of them. They purport to detoxify the body, and thus relieve you of your ailments, including allergies. But do they deliver on their promises?

"Health begins in the colon," say proponents of a therapeutic modality known as colonic irrigation. How true is that statement? Colonic irrigation, also known as colon cleansing, formerly known as "high colonic," is a detoxification therapy whose treatments aim to free the body from toxins and pollutants that are said to have leaked into the bloodstream, weakening the immune system so as to render it susceptible to antigens, thus leaving you wide open for allergic reactions. During treatments, a special colon irrigation machine pumps warm, purified water into the lower bowel to loosen and remove the built-up feces that supposedly are clinging to the walls of your intestines.

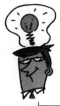

Bet You Didn't Know

In early times, the procedure we now know as colonic irrigation or colon therapy was performed in rivers, using a hollow reed.

Colon therapy has its roots in Egypt, Greece, and India, where enemas were first used centuries ago to cleanse the body of disease. By the 1890s, this therapy had reached American shores, and thousands of enthusiasts flocked to newly opened spas that advertised health and rejuvenation through "high colonic" enemas.

Getting On With It

How does colonic irrigation flush toxins from the bowel? A small tube is inserted 5½ inches into your rectum. The tube is attached to a plastic hose and connected to a colon irrigation machine. This device will slowly fill the five-foot length of your colon with warm water. The water causes the muscles lining your colon to expand and contract, forcing out all that crappy sludge you've been holding inside, through an evacuation tube. The procedure will be repeated until a total of 20 to 30 gallons of water has been flushed through your bowel.

And now, peristalsis is restored to your system, your bowel movements improve, your blood is freshly cleansed of toxins, your immune system is in optimum shape, your body is healthy—and, we hope, you are feeling great.

A variation of colonic irrigation is the coffee enema, a technique devised some 60 or more years ago by Dr. Max Gerson. Today, this form of colon therapy is still practiced at the Gerson Clinic in Tijuana, Mexico, and in 17 other clinics. The caffeine in the enemas is claimed to stimulate the production of bile from the liver, and thus improve gastrointestinal problems, including food allergy reactions. Despite glowing testimonials, this therapy has not been clinically tested through peer review.

> **Skulls and Bones**
>
> Laxatives and enemas are sometimes used as part of colonic therapy. Overuse can damage your colon. Also, large quantities of water can stretch the bowel so that it no longer functions properly. Avoid colon therapy if you have Crohn's disease, diverticulitis, hemorrhoids, tumors of the large intestine or rectum, or ulcerative colitis.

So Prove It, Already

Now the downside of both colon cleansing and coffee enemas. Mainstream medicine doesn't buy it. Doctors maintain that there is no evidence that our diets produce toxins in the bowel, or that fecal matter clings to the intestinal walls, or that accumulated feces turns poisonous. Instead, doctors recommend you try a high-fiber diet and increase fluid intake if you have a problem with elimination.

Whether or not a colonic irrigation procedure is going to help your food allergy symptoms is problematic. One thing it may accomplish is relief of stress and bloating. Aside from the foregoing, these treatments could pose a risk of chemical imbalance, enzyme deficiency, weakness, a perforated intestine or bowel dysfunction, infections, and other problems, including alternating constipation and diarrhea. Nevertheless, this treatment has its advocates who swear by it, and claim it helps relieve their allergy symptoms. Only you—and your physician—can decide.

> **Bet You Didn't Know**
>
> The most famous early colonic therapist was John Harvey Kellogg, founder of the eponymous cereal company in Battle Creek, Michigan. Kellogg's sanitarium treated over 40,000 patients.

Okay to Chelate?

Chelation's goal is to reduce or remove heavy metal poisoning from your system. It can remove calcium, an ingredient in arterial plaque, with a chemical called ethylene-diaminetetracetic acid (EDTA). This substance is administered through an intravenous (IV) needle inserted in a vein in your finger or hand. Some chelation practitioners claim the procedure can help "cure" allergies of any kind. This assertion is unfounded and unproven.

Bet You Didn't Know ____

EDTA was first used to remove calcium from pipes and boilers, then found effective for treating workers with lead poisoning. Doctors noticed that patients treated with EDTA for lead poisoning reported less pain from angina and an increase in energy. Medical proponents of chelation began believing chelation could be useful for many different medical conditions.

Skulls and Bones ____

Chelation treatments are not advised for anything other than metal poisoning. If you are pregnant or have kidney damage, liver disease, or a brain tumor, avoid chelation. Avoid it also if you have heart disease or cancer.

The term *chelation* comes from the Greek word *chele*, meaning "claw." Like a claw, EDTA grabs the metals in your bloodstream and carries them through your system to be excreted in your urine.

Most physicians disagree with chelation's theories, saying that chelation is deemed effective only for removing heavy metals from the bloodstream, but that beyond that, claims are unsubstantiated by peer review. Although chelation proponents assert that the technique relieves a variety of physical complaints, including the varied symptoms of food allergies, such benefits have not been demonstrated by any well-designed clinical trials.

Further, as an allergy sufferer, you should know that excessive use of chelation has been known to cause problems such as anemia, blood clots, bone marrow damage, fever, insulin shock, irregular heartbeat, joint pain, low blood pressure, painful urination, and stroke.

Before starting chelation, you'll be given a thorough physical exam. When questioned about your health and that of family members, be sure to mention any allergies and list all the medications you're taking.

Cell Therapy Treatments

Traditional cell therapy claims that when injected into a human patient, animal fetal cells will automatically travel to the corresponding human organ or gland and revitalize it. Animal cells or extracts injected into the human bloodstream are said to improve the recipient's health, relieve pain, inflammation, and other symptoms of food allergies, and enhance youth. The method was pioneered in the 1930s by Dr. Paul Niehans at his clinic in Vevey, Switzerland. Many world leaders as well as the rich and famous have received these treatments, including the late Charlie Chaplin (who fathered children when well into his 80s), Charles de Gaulle, Konrad Adenauer, Pope Pius XII, Gloria Swanson, and among the living, film stars Elizabeth Taylor and George Hamilton.

Cells used in the therapy are usually taken from unborn sheep, pigs, or other farm animals. (People for Ethical Treatment of Animals, or PETA, would not approve.) Originally, fresh live cells were prepared by combining the sacrificed animals' tissues or glands with a saline solution. Today freeze-dried cells are used, or antibodies produced from the cells.

A more developed version of cell therapy treatments uses antibodies. Injections are produced by administering the cells to an animal, whose immune system then manufactures antibodies in response. These antibodies are then harvested from the animal's blood, purified, and administered to the patient.

Although cell therapy is practiced at spas and clinics in Germany, the Bahamas, Switzerland, and Mexico, the treatments are banned in the United States due to the danger of infection and allergic reaction.

You should also know that cell therapy is expensive (often several thousand dollars), but is cheaper in Mexico than elsewhere. It is unlikely your insurance will cover these treatments. Be sure to get everything in writing so you know exactly what your total cost will be.

> **Skulls and Bones**
>
> Cell therapy is not recommended for those with kidney and liver disease, infections, and inflammatory diseases such as ulcerative colitis. Fatigue may result and endure for two weeks following injections. There is also the danger of allergic reaction, and your immune system could reject the material.

The Power of Suggestion

Through the power of suggestion, hypnosis can relieve all types of pain, and may be helpful for anxiety, tension, depression, nausea and vomiting, and other allergy symptoms as well. Proponents say hypnosis can "trick" the body into healing itself of any and all negative conditions, including symptoms of food allergies.

Hypnotherapy uses the induction of a trancelike state to reach the unconscious level of the mind. In a relaxed hypnotic state, receptive to positive suggestion, you can learn to react differently to pain and discomfort associated with your allergy symptoms.

The modern version of hypnotherapy began in the eighteenth century, when Austrian physician Franz Anton Mesmer, believing illness to represent imbalance in the body's magnetic forces, attempted to cure disease by animal magnetism. Today hypnotherapy is medically accepted as an adjunctive treatment to ease troublesome symptoms of allergy.

No one is sure how hypnosis works. Some scientists speculate it prompts the brain to release enkephalins and endorphins that can change the way we perceive pain and other physical symptoms; other scientists believe hypnosis may act through the unconscious.

One of hypnotherapy's greatest benefits is its ability to reduce our reaction to stress. If you believe, as many physicians and psychologists do, that the mind has an impact on our physical well-being, then you can see how tension, anxiety, and depression undermine health, while a positive attitude can reinforce the immune system, enabling it to better fight health problems. When negative patterns are broken, your entire body feels healthier.

Are You a Candidate?

Hypnosis doesn't work for everybody. Roughly one person in ten can't be hypnotized. You can be tested to see if you'll make a good candidate. Some of the tests that will let you know are the Stanford Hypnotic Susceptibility Scales; the Barber Suggestibility Scale; the Harvard Group Scale of Hypnotic Susceptibility; the eye-roll test; the light test; and the lemon test.

Several techniques can be used to put you into a hypnotic trance, the most common of which are: asking you to watch a moving object such as a pendulum as it swings back and forth; suggesting in a monotonous, soothing voice that your eyes are getting so heavy you can't keep them open; telling you to concentrate on the therapist's voice as he or she gives you instructions; and having you count backward slowly from 100 to 0.

As you slip into a trance, you'll feel increasingly relaxed. As your conscious mind gives up its hold, your surroundings seem to recede. Concentrate your attention on something pleasant. Negative thoughts will clear from your mind as you focus on the suggestions your therapist gives you, perhaps to make pain disappear, or to make you less susceptible to the stress component of allergy symptoms.

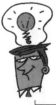

Bet You Didn't Know

British ophthalmologist James Braid coined the term *hypnosis,* after the Greek word for "sleep."

At the end of the session, the hypnotist will suggest how wonderful you'll feel when you wake, and will order you to wake up refreshed, healthy, and hopefully symptom-free.

Do It Yourself

You can hypnotize yourself. Get comfortable and relax. Let your muscles go limp, and feel the tension flowing out of your body.

Focus your mind, either through gazing at an object or picture, or imagining yourself in a quiet, restful place. Concentrate as you breathe deeply and slowly. You may repeat a word or phrase, such as a mantra; you may wish to repeat the mantra "Om" out loud to induce the trance state.

Once you've achieved a hypnotic state, you can instruct yourself how you want to feel, or you may listen to a tape on which you have pre-recorded a positive message. You will wake by counting slowly from 10 back to zero. Tell yourself you're going to awaken feeling fantastic and that you are in perfect health.

Timely Tip

You can learn self-hypnosis from audio and videotapes. Professionals who specialize in hypnosis advise also taking lessons from a qualified hypnotherapist.

Hyping Hyperthermia and Other Hypes

Hyperthermia assumes that heat, as administered in a sauna, steam, or Turkish bath, can remove toxins from the body and make you healthy again. Hyperthermia, doctors agree, can relieve pain. Adherents also claim it can reduce inflammation and other symptoms caused by food allergies.

When undertaking hyperthermia, observe time limits, because excessive hyperthermia can be dangerous. Limit sessions in a Turkish bath or steam room to 20 minutes. If you take a sauna, you will need to take a cold shower every 5 to 10 minutes. And remember to drink plenty of water.

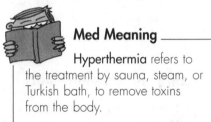

Med Meaning

Hyperthermia refers to the treatment by sauna, steam, or Turkish bath, to remove toxins from the body.

If your food allergy manifests as hives, eczema, or asthma, you should double-check with your allergist to make sure this treatment is not contraindicated, and your heart specialist if you have problems with high blood pressure or heart problems.

Hot Stuff, Wet Towels

Claims for hot fomentation include solving problems of depression, anxiety, pain, and some allergic symptoms, such as bloating, gas, respiratory distress, and others. This form of therapy combines application of hot and cold wet towels with the administration of electrical stimulation.

Constitutional hydrotherapy treatments are similar to hot fomentation, minus the electrical stimulator. Constitutional hydrotherapy originated nearly 100 years ago. Proponents today believe that alternate applications of heat and cold can increase the body's white blood cell count and enhance its ability to fight disease. Should you feel worse rather than better following treatments, it is claimed that the negative reaction is creating a healing crisis; your body is throwing off harmful toxins; you have to get worse before you get better to effect a cure.

Muds R Us

A similar technique is used, particularly in European spas, with local radioactive muds. Over the past couple of decades, these treatments have also come into vogue at a number of spas in the United States, although U.S. spas don't usually claim their muds are radioactive.

Treatments in which the body and face are covered with special hot muds are helpful for pain. The treatments do relax and rejuvenate, and they also enervate, so that you will need to rest afterwards. If you take a series of treatments, you will get used to them so that you won't be as tired afterwards. These treatments are said to ease tension and soothe allergy symptoms, including those caused by food allergies. Mud treatments are said to relieve nasal congestion, bloating, gas, constipation, and skin eruptions.

In many spas, particularly in Europe, an on-site physician's approval is first necessary before you are allowed to take the treatments. Patients with heart and other serious medical problems, for instance, are denied clearance.

Getting Along Swimmingly

Hydrotherapy assumes that water treatments can detoxify and restore the body to health. Watsu, an aquatic deep-tissue massage, helps pain and tension. In this form of therapy, a therapist floats a patient through the water in a sequence of movements. Watsu, created at the School of Shiatsu and Massage in Harbin Springs, California, is recommended to relieve stiffness and tension. It may help relieve symptoms of food allergies such as bloating, constipation, gas, diarrhea, and others.

Although aquatic physical therapy is recognized by many insurance providers for specific types of rehabilitation, allergy symptoms are unlikely to qualify for insurance benefits. Called hydrotherapy in Europe, this therapy is recommended for patients who experience pain during physical therapy outside water, or whose rehabilitation will be helped in a water environment.

Procedures include whirlpool baths and aquatic therapy in a swimming pool. The treatments relax and reduce stress, tension, and anxiety, thus perhaps improving certain types of allergies, such as those previously mentioned. A modification of this type of exercise—swimming you do on your own—will relax you and help you feel better.

Skulls and Bones

Aquatic physical therapy is contraindicated if you have inner ear problems, a disorder of the spine, an acute injury, or unstable joint. Constitutional hydrotherapy and hot fomentation are ill advised if you suffer from kidney disease, asthma, a weak heart or bleeding disorder, an organ transplant, metal implants, or a pacemaker.

The Least You Need to Know

♦ Extreme caution is advised if you are considering colon cleansing (colonic irrigation) or coffee enemas; don't count on them curing your allergies, either. Beware of the possible serious complications.

♦ Chelation will clear out toxic metals, but has not been proven to be effective in other cases.

♦ Cell therapy advocates claim it has worked for them; it can be dangerous and is expensive.

♦ Hypnotherapy works and can reduce stress, helping ease allergy symptoms and your reactions to them.

Resources

This appendix lists organizations and other resources that provide further information for people suffering from food allergies.

Organizations

Allergy and Asthma Network—Mothers of Asthmatics, Inc.
2751 Prosperity Avenue, Suite 150
Fairfax, VA 22031
1-800-878-4403 or 703-385-4403
Fax: 703-573-7794
www.aanma.org
Newsletter: *The MA Report*

American Academy of Allergy, Asthma and Immunology
611 East Wells Street
Milwaukee, WI 53202
1-800-822-2762 or 414-272-6071
www.aaaai.org

American Academy of Dermatology
930 N. Meacham Road
Schaumburg, IL 60173
1-888-462-DERM
www.aad.org

American College of Allergy, Asthma and Immunology
85 West Algonquin Road, Suite 550
Arlington Heights, IL 60005
708-427-1200
www.allergy.mcg.edu

American Dietetic Association
216 W. Jackson Boulevard
Chicago, IL 60606-6995
1-800-877-1600
www.eatright.org

Anaphylaxis Foundation of Canada
Suite 2054
3080 Younge Street
Toronto, Ontario M4N 3N1
Canada
416-926-7697
Fax: 416-926-4491

Anaphylaxis Network of Canada
PO Box 57524, 1500 Royal York Road
Etobicoke, Ontario M9P 3B6
Canada
416-785-5666
Fax: 416-243-7733

**Asthma and Allergy Foundation
of America**
1125 15th Street NW, Suite 502
Washington, DC 20005
1-800-727-8462 or 202-466-7643
Fax: 202-466-8940
www.aafa.org
Newsletter: *The Asthma and Allergy
Advance*

**Food Allergy Anaphylaxis Network
(FAAN)**
10400 Eaton Place, Suite 107
Fairfax, VA 22030-2208
703-691-3179
Fax: 703-691-2713
www.foodallergy.org

La Leche League International
9616 Minneapolis Avenue
Franklin Park, IL 60131
312-455-7730
www.lalecheleague.org

Medic Alert Foundation
2323 Colorado Avenue
Turlock, CA 95382-2018
1-800-432-5378
www.medicalert.org

**National Arthritis, Musculoskeletal
and Skin Diseases Information
Clearinghouse**
One AMS Circle
Bethesda, MD 20892-3675
301-495-4484
www.nih.gov/niams/

**National Digestive Diseases
Information Clearinghouse**
Box NDDIC
Bethesda, MD 20892
301-654-3810
www.niddk.nih.gov/health/digest/
pubs/lactose/lactose.htm
www.niddk.nih.gov/health/digest/
pubs/celiac/index.htm

**National Eczema Association for
Science and Education**
4460 Redwood Highway, Suite 16-D
San Rafael, CA 94903-1953
1-800-818-7546
www.nationaleczema.org/home.html

**National Institute of Allergy and
Infectious Diseases**
Building 31, Room 7A-50
31 Center Drive MSC 2520
Bethesda, MD 20892-2520
301-496-5717
www.niaid.nih.gov/

U.S. Department of Agriculture
Food and Nutrition Information
Center
301-436-7725
www.nalusda.gov/fnic/index.html

Websites

Allergy, Asthma and Immunology Online
allergy.mcg.edu

American Academy of Allergy Asthma & Immunology
www.aaaai.org

American Academy of Pediatrics
www.aap.org/

American Medical Association
www.ama-assn.org

Anaphylaxis Canada
www.anaphylaxis.org

CDC Travelers' Health
www.cdc.gov/travel/

Center for Healthcare Information
www.cmrg.com/

Clinical Trials.gov
www.clinicaltrials.gov

CultureMed
www.sunyit.edu/library/html/culturemed/

Food Anaphylaxis Education
www.faemi.org

Food and Drug Administration
www.fda.gov

Mothers of Children Having Allergies (MOCHA)
www.mochallergies.org

National Center for Complementary and Alternative Medicine
nccam.nih.gov

National Institute of Health
www.niaid.nih.gov

National Library of Medicine's MEDLINEplus
www.nlm.nih.gov

NLM's Toxnet and Toxtown
toxnet.nlm.nih.gov
toxtown.nlm.nih.gov

Selected Travel Resources

Clements International
Washington, DC
1-800-872-0067 or 202-872-0060
info@clements.com
www.clements.com

Gateway
Seabury & Smith
Washington, DC
1-800-282-4495 or 202-457-7707
gateway.dc@seabury.com

Health Quest Travel, Inc.
Wexford, PA
1-888-899-3633
healthquesttravel.com
HQT@HealthQuestTravel.com

InsureMyTrip.com
Commack, NY
1-800-487-4722
info@insuremytrip.com
insuremytrip.com

Medical Travel, Inc.
5184 Majorca Club Drive
Boca Raton, FL 33486
1-800-778-7953
info@medicaltravel.org

Mercury International Travel
Frances C. Wollach-Staros, CTA
630 Fifth Avenue
New York, NY 10111
1-800-847-3738, ext. 641
fwollach@merctravel.com
www.perfectmatchusa.com

Wellontheroad.com
Healthcare Information for
the International Traveler
wellontheroad.com

Worldwide Assistance
Washington, DC
1-800-777-8710, ext. 417

Adverse Food Reactions and Their Causes

Adverse symptoms that occur after eating foods are not always due to allergy or intolerance. You should be aware of other possible causes. The following lists show various other causes that can affect your body and might be mistaken for food allergy or food intolerance.

Gastrointestinal Disorders

Symptom	Condition	Example
Vomiting	Gastrointestinal	Gastroesophageal reflux
		Obstruction
		Peptic ulcer disease
		Hepatitis
		Pancreatitis
		Acute gastroenteritis
		Motility disturbances
	Psychogenic	Anorexia nervosa
		Psychosocial vomiting

Gastrointestinal Disorders   (continued)

Symptom	Condition	Example
Extra intestinal	Metabolic	Reye's syndrome Lead poisoning
	Toxic	Drug toxicity, ingestion Infection Meningitis, encephalitis Increased intracranial pressure Tumor Trauma
Diarrhea	Infections	Viral Bacterial Chronic inflammation
	Abnormality of anatomy	Intestinal obstruction Chronic constipation
	Inadequate pancreatic function	Cystic fibrosis
	Abnormality of the intestinal lining	Celiac disease Cow's milk or soy protein intolerance
	Miscellaneous	Irritable bowel Hyperthyroidism

Illnesses That Mimic Food Allergy

Type	Illness
Structural abnormality	Hiatal hernia Pyloric stenosis Acid reflux
Enzyme deficiency	Lactase deficiency Lactose intolerance
Malignancy	Stomach cancer
Other	Cystic fibrosis Gall bladder disease Peptic ulcer

Contaminants and Additives

Contaminant/Additive	Example
Flavorings and preservatives	MSG Nitrites/nitrates Sodium metabisulfite (such as in red wine)
Toxins	Bacterial-clostridium botulinum, Staphylococcus aureus Fungal-aflatoxins, ergot (infection on wheat)
Seafood	Scombroid poisoning (tuna, mackerel) Ciguatera poisoning (barracuda, snapper) Saxitoxin (shellfish)
Infectious organisms	Bacteria Parasites Viruses
Accidental contaminants	Pesticides Heavy metals Antibiotics
Pharmacologic agents	Caffeine Histamine Serotinin (bananas and tomatoes) Tyramine (cheeses, pickled herring) Alcohol

Foods That Liberate Mediators from Mast Cells

- Alcohol
- Chocolate
- Crustaceans
- Egg whites
- Fish
- Papaya
- Pineapple
- Strawberries
- Tomatoes

Foods That Are Naturally Toxic

Type	Food
Unsafe foods	Amanita mushrooms
	Foxglove/digitalis
	Puffer fish/salamanders
	Rhubarb leaves
	Beet leaves
	Sorrel
Unsafe when eaten under special conditions	Raw red beans
	Green potatoes
	Lima bean varieties
Unsafe when eaten in excessive quantities	Lima beans
	Cassava root
	Millet/sorghum
	Apricot and peach pits
	Bitter almond
Unsafe when eaten in large amounts by people with metabolic problems	Cabbage family
	Turnips
	Soybeans
	Watercress
	Radishes
	Grape seed
	Mustard
Natural foods that give gastrointestinal symptoms	Cucumbers
	Beans
	Berries

Glossary

acid reflux   A condition in which stomach acid refluxes up from the stomach into the esophagus.

acupressure   Acupuncture without needles, acupressure helps heal illness by applying deep finger pressure at points located along the fourteen meridians where the body's vital energy or Qi flows, connecting vital organs throughout the body.

acupuncture   A procedure using acupuncture needles along meridian lines to help control pain and help control other medical problems.

adrenalin   *See* epinephrine.

Allegra   A nonsedating, highly selective H1 receptor antagonist of histamine with no atropinelike actions.

allergen   Antigen responsible for producing allergic reactions by inducing IgE formation; substance that triggers an allergic reaction.

allergic rhinitis   Inflammation of the mucous membranes of the nose due to an allergic response; also known as hay fever.

allergist   A physician specializing in the treatment of allergies.

allergy   Inappropriate or exaggerated reaction of the immune system to substances that, in the majority of people, cause no symptoms.

allergy skin test   Injection of a small quantity of an allergen into the skin; used to figure out what allergens trigger a person's allergic response.

anaphylaxis   Sudden, severe, potentially life-threatening allergic reaction caused by food allergies, insect stings, or medications. Symptoms can include hives, swelling (especially of the lips and face), difficulty breathing (either because of swelling in the throat or an asthmatic reaction), vomiting, diarrhea, cramping, and a drop in blood pressure.

anti-inflammatory drugs   Drugs that reduce the symptoms and signs of inflammation.

antibody   A complex protein that is manufactured by lymphocytes to neutralize or destroy an antigen or foreign protein. Many types of antibodies are protective; however, inappropriate or excessive formation of antibodies may lead to illness. It is also described as a molecule produced by B cells in response to stimulation by an antigen.

antigen   A substance that can trigger an immune response, resulting in production of an antibody as part of the body's defense against infection and disease. Many antigens are foreign proteins (those not found naturally in the body). An allergen is a special type of antigen that causes an IgE antibody response.

antigen-binding site   Part of an immunoglobulin molecule that binds antigen specifically.

antihistamine drugs   A group of drugs that block the effects of histamine, a chemical released in body fluids during an allergic reaction.

asthma   A chronic, inflammatory lung disease characterized by recurrent breathing problems. People with asthma have acute episodes when the air passages in their lungs get narrower, and breathing becomes more difficult. Sometimes episodes of asthma are triggered by allergens, although infection, exercise, cold air, and other factors are also important triggers.

atopic   From the Greek *a-topos*, meaning "without a place." Atopic conditions of asthma, hay fever, and eczema (atopic dermatitis) were originally classified as "strange diseases."

atopic dermatitis   Eczema.

atopy   Describing IgE-mediated anaphylactic responses in humans, usually genetically determined.

autoimmunity (autoallergy)   An immune response to "self" tissues or components. Such an immune response may have pathological consequences leading to autoimmune diseases.

Ayurveda   Indian medical system, meaning knowledge of life.

B lymphocyte (B cell)   Precursors of antibody-forming plasma cells; these cells carry immunoglobulin and class II MHC (major histocompatibility complex) antigens on their surfaces.

basophil   Polymorphonuclear leukocyte whose basophils granules contain heparin, histamine, and other vasoactive amines. Within tissues, these cells are known as mast cells, q.v.

blood brain barrier   Describing the lining capillaries of the central nervous system (CNS). Any medication that crosses the blood brain barrier has an effect on the function of the CNS. In the case of antihistamines, the effects are to cause drowsiness and prevent nausea.

board-certified allergist   Doctor who is trained in internal medicine and/or pediatrics, in addition to which he or she is trained in adult and pediatric allergy, asthma, and clinical immunology. He or she must be tested and certified by the specialty organization.

bronchitis   Inflammation of the mucous membranes of the bronchial tubes, causing a persistent cough that produces considerable quantities of sputum (phlegm).

bronchodilators   A group of drugs that widen the airways in the lungs.

celiac disease   Also called celiac sprue or gluten sensitive enteropathy. It is a sensitivity to gluten, a wheat protein. Individuals with this disease must avoid gluten-containing grains, which include all forms of wheat, oats, barley, and rye.

cell-mediated immunity (CMI)   An immune reaction mediated by T cells; in contrast to humoral immunity, which is antibody mediated. Also referred to as delayed-type hypersensitivity.

cirrhosis   End-stage liver disease with widespread damage to the cells, nodules, and scarring. This is associated with failure of liver function and blockage of blood flow to the liver.

citrus   A type of food such as oranges or grapefruit.

classical homeopathy   Use of a single remedy prescribed according to the individual's presentation and history.

colic   Cramping, pain, and bloating as symptoms of abdominal problem.

complement   A series of serum proteins involved in the mediation of immune reactions. The complement cascade is triggered classically by the interaction of antibody with specific antigen.

complex homeopathy   More than one remedy used concurrently.

contact dermatitis   An inflammation of the skin, or a rash caused by contact with various substances of a chemical, animal, or vegetable nature. The reaction may be an immunologic response or a direct toxic effect of the substance. Among the more common causes of a contact dermatitis reaction are detergents left on washed clothes, nickel (in watch straps, bracelets, necklaces, and the fastenings on underclothes), chemicals in rubber gloves and condoms, certain cosmetics, plants such as poison ivy, and topical medications.

Coombs' test   A test named for its originator, R.R.A. Coombs, used to detect non-agglutinating antibodies on red blood cells by addition of an anti-immunoglobulin antibody.

corticosteroid drugs   A group of anti-inflammatory drugs similar to the natural corticosteroid hormones produced by the cortex of the adrenal glands. Among the disorders that often improve with corticosteroid treatment are asthma, allergic rhinitis, eczema, and rheumatoid arthritis.

cortisone   Glucocorticoid $C_{21}H_{28}O_5$ produced naturally in small amounts by the adrenal cortex and administered in the form of the acetate of its synthetic form especially as replacement therapy for deficient adrenocortical secretion and as an anti-inflammatory agent.

cradle cap or **seborrheic dermatitis**   A scaly eruption that involves the diaper area and scalp.

crustacean   A type of shellfish with a soft shell.

cytotoxic test   A diagnostic test said to be able to identify allergy to food by the reaction of the food when added to a preparation of blood cells.

dairy products   Foods derived from cow's milk.

dander   A term used to describe the superficial layer of skin in an animal.

decongestant   Medication used to decrease swelling of a tissue by causing constriction of the blood vessels in the tissue.

degranulation   The process of losing granules; the process by which cytoplasmic granules (as of mast cells) release their contents.

delayed type hypersensitivity (DTH)   T cell-mediated reaction to antigen, which takes 24 to 48 hours to develop fully, and which involves release of lymphokines and recruitment of monocytes and macrophages. Also called cell-mediated immunity.

dermatographism   A weltlike reaction of the skin in the form or pattern of the stroking or pressure on the skin. A person can form a letter or name, which appears as a white or blanched line followed by a red area. For this reason it has been called autographism. The weltlike area will disappear soon after the irritation. This condition is also known as dermatographia as well as dermographism, the skin you can write on.

digestive system   The group of organs that breaks down food into chemical components that the body can absorb and use for energy, and for building and repairing cells and tissues.

double-blind cross-over   A test procedure using both known antigen and placebo. The individual is given each in random order. Neither the patient nor the physician knows what order is being used until the test is completed. The patient's reaction to each separate test material is noted.

dust mites   A microscopic organism found in the skin and hair of people. This can be an allergen or antigen.

eczema   An inflammation of the skin, usually causing itching and sometimes accompanied by crusting, scaling, or blisters. A type of eczema often made worse by allergen exposure is termed "atopic dermatitis."

EDS or EDT testing   A form of modified electroacupuncture. It is an unorthodox technique to diagnose allergies and other diseases.

electrodermal testing   Measures electric charge on an acupuncture point and is a form of unconventional testing for allergies.

elimination challenge   A form of testing in which a suspected food is removed from the diet for a specified period of time and then reintroduced to see if this causes symptoms. This should be done with the supervision of a physician.

endoscopy   A medical procedure in which a device like a telescope is used, allowing the physician to look into a cavity of the body. In the case of acid reflux, the doctor can look down into the esophagus to see what, if any, damage has been done, and exactly where in the esophagus it's occurring.

enzyme   A protein that acts to start chemical changes in other substances while it remains unchanged during the process. Most enzymes are named by adding the letters "ase" to the name of the material it works on, the substance activated, or the type of reaction.

enzyme-linked immunosorbent assay (ELISA)   An assay in which an enzyme is linked to an antibody and a colored substrate is used to measure the activity of bound enzyme and, hence, the amount of bound antibody.

eosinophil   Polymorphonuclear leukocyte with large eosinophilic (i.e., red) cytoplasmic granules.

epinephrine   A naturally occurring hormone, also called adrenaline. It is one of two chemicals (the other is norepinephrine) released by the adrenal gland. Epinephrine increases the speed and force of heartbeats and, thereby, the work that can be done by the heart. It dilates the airways to improve breathing and narrows blood vessels in the skin and intestine so that an increased flow of blood reaches the muscles and allows them to cope with the demands of exercise. Epinephrine has been produced synthetically as a drug since 1900. It remains the drug of choice for treatment of anaphylaxis.

EpiPen   A spring-loaded syringe containing epinephrine.

FDA   Food and Drug Administration.

food additive   A substance added to a processed food that is usually artificially produced.

food allergen   A protein within food that usually is not broken down either by cooking or by stomach acids or enzymes and may cause an allergic reactions.

food allergy   A reaction in the body the acts through IgE.

food diary   A log that notes all foods eaten each day.

food intolerance   An adverse food-induced reaction that does not involve the immune system. Lactose intolerance is an example.

GALT   Gut Associated Lymphoid Tissue. Protects the body from potential bacterial invaders. It is composed of lymphocyte white blood cells, spread out in at least three locations.

gastrocrome   Medication that is cromolyn sodium and used as a mast cell stabilizer so that the mast cell does not break down and release mediators.

gastrointestinal tract   A term for the digestive tract.

genes   Protein structures that act as a unit of heredity. They are arranged like a bead on a string or filament. Specific genes are always found in the same location (locus). They direct or act as a pattern for forming an enzyme or other proteins.

GERD   Gastroesophageal reflux disease.

geriatrics   A medical specialty that treats the elderly.

gluten sensitive enteropathy   Also called celiac sprue or celiac disease. It is a sensitivity to gluten, a wheat protein. Individuals with this disease must avoid gluten-containing grains, which include all forms of wheat, oats, barley, and rye.

granulocytes   White blood cells whose interior liquid contains granules that contain enzymes capable of killing microorganisms and breaking down debris they ingest. Granulocytes include the neutrophil, the eosinophil and basophil cells, the neutrophil being the most abundant of these immune cells, comprising 50 to 70 percent of the total white cell count. Neutrophils are phagocytic, meaning they gobble up any foreign bacteria they come across.

hay fever *See* rhinitis.

heartburn A burning sensation that starts behind the breastbone and moves from under the breastbone toward the neck.

helper T cells A class of T cells which help trigger B cells to make antibodies against thymus-dependent antigens. Helper T cells also help generate cytotoxic T cells.

hemodialysis A medical procedure to remove wastes or toxins from the blood and adjust fluid and electrolyte imbalances by utilizing rates at which substances diffuse through a semipermeable membrane; the process of removing blood from an artery (as of a kidney patient), purifying it by dialysis, adding vital substances, and returning it to a vein.

hepatitis An inflammation of the liver due to viral infection or toxic agents.

hernia A protrusion of an organ or tissue through an opening in its surrounding walls, especially in the abdominal region. Another word used for this is a rupture.

hiatal hernia When part of the stomach moves upward through the esophageal hiatus or opening in the diaphragm and causes digestive discomfort.

hiatus An opening or aperture (like the one on your camera).

Hippocrates Greek physician, called the father of medicine, practiced circa 400 B.C.E., and wrote the Hippocratic Oath.

histamine A chemical present in cells throughout the body that is released during an allergic reaction. It is one of the substances responsible for the symptoms of inflammation and is the major reason for running of the nose, sneezing, and itching in allergic rhinitis. It also stimulates production of acid by the stomach and narrows the bronchi or airways in the lungs.

hives (urticaria) An allergic reaction of the skin consisting of itchy, raised white lumps surrounded by an area of red inflammation.

hyper High.

hypersensitivity State of reactivity to an antigen that is greater than normal for the antigenic challenge; hypersensitivity is the same as allergy and denotes a deleterious outcome rather than a protective one.

hyperthermia   Treatment by sauna, steam, or Turkish bath to remove toxins from the body.

hypo   Low.

idiosyncrasy   An abnormal reaction to a drug or a chemical or opposite response.

IgA   Immunoglobulin usually associated with digestive tract secretions.

IgE   Immunoglobulin usually associated with allergic reactions.

immediate-type hypersensitivity   Hypersensitivity tissue reaction occurring within minutes after the interaction of antigen and antibody.

immune complex   An antigen bound to an antibody.

immune system   A collection of cells and proteins that works to protect the body from potentially harmful, infectious microorganisms (microscopic life forms) such as bacteria, viruses, and fungi. The immune system plays a role in the control of cancer and other diseases but also is the culprit in the phenomena of allergies, hypersensitivity, and the rejection of transplanted organs, tissues, and medical implants.

immunogen   A substance capable of inducing an immune response (as well as reacting with the products of an immune response). Compare with antigen.

immunogenetics   A study that explains our inheritance and our development.

immunoglobulin (Ig)   A general term for all antibody molecules. Each Ig unit is made up of two heavy chains and two light chains and has two antigen-binding sites.

immunoglobulin E (IgE)   A type of protein called an antibody that circulates through the blood. Immunoglobin E is formed to protect the body from infection, which attaches to mast cells in the respiratory and intestinal tracts and may cause allergic rhinitis, asthma, or eczema.

immunoglobulins   Antibodies or proteins found in blood and tissue fluids produced by cells of the immune system to bind to substances in the body that are recognized as foreign antigens. Immunoglobulins sometimes bind to antigens that are not necessarily a threat to health and provoke an allergic reaction.

immunotherapy (allergy shots)   A treatment for people who are allergic to pollen, house dust mites, fungi, or stinging insect venom; involves injections of gradually increasing doses of the substance, or allergen, to which the person is allergic. The incremental increases of the allergen cause the immune system to become less sensitive to the substance, which reduces the symptoms of an allergy when the substance is encountered in the future.

inflammation   Redness, swelling, heat, and pain in a tissue due to chemical or physical injury, infection, or allergic reactions in the nose, lungs, and skin.

intradermal   Within the substance of the skin and below the cutis.

iridology   The study of the iris of the eye, the exposed nerve endings which are connected to the brain. It is said that a trained iridologist can tell genetic inheritance, congestive and irritative zones and their various interreactions within the body.

J chain (joining chain)   Polypeptide involved in the polymerization of immunoglobulin molecules IgM and I.

lactose intolerance   A condition that occurs when a person cannot break down the sugar in cow's milk (lactose). It cannot be absorbed, often causing symptoms of bloating, abdominal pain, diarrhea, or constipation.

law of similars ("like cures like")   Homeopathy's fundamental concept, which alleges that (a) any pharmacologically active agent will create a characteristic set of symptoms when administered to healthy individuals; (b) sick individuals will display a specific set of symptoms that express their illness; and (c) administration of the "similar" medicine to the sick patient will initiate a curative response.

lectin   Latin for "choosing." The lectin is very specific for certain carbohydrate molecules on the mast cell surface. If it does not match one, it will not attach.

legume   A type of food such as pea, bean, and peanut.

lichenification   Thickening of the epidermal layer of skin.

lipid   Fat-soluble. Substances that are extracted from or gotten out of animal and vegetable cells by certain solvents. The building blocks of lipids are called fatty acids. These appear in long chains of carbon molecules, which are 14 to 24 carbons in length.

LPR   Laryngopharyngeal reflux, backflow of stomach contents into the throat, the larynx, the pharynx, and the esophagus.

lymphocyte   Any of a group of white blood cells of crucial importance to the adaptive part of the body's immune system. The adaptive portion of the immune system mounts a tailor-made defense when dangerous invading organisms penetrate the body's general defenses.

lymphokines   Soluble substances secreted by lymphocytes, which have a variety of effects on lymphocytes and other cell types.

macrophage   A large phagocytic cell of the mononuclear series found within tissues. Properties include phagocytosis, and antigen presentation to T cells.

mast cell stabilizer   Substance such as cromolyn sodium that prevents the breakdown of mast cells.

mast cells   Cells which synthesize and store histamines, found in most body tissues, particularly just below the epithelial surfaces in serous cavities, and around blood vessels. In an allergic response, an allergen stimulates the release of antibodies, which attach themselves to mast cells.

mediator   Substance that plays a part in the production of inflammation.

memory   Active state of immunity to a specific antigen, such that a second encounter with that antigen leads to a larger and more rapid response.

milk allergy   An immune system reaction involving IgE to milk.

mollusk   A type of shellfish with a hard shell, such as a clam or oyster.

monocyte   A large, circulating white cell, 2–10 percent of total white cells, phagocytic, indented nucleus. It migrates to tissues, where it is known as a macrophage.

Munchausen syndrome   A situation where a person pretends to have any number of symptoms so that he or she can be hospitalized, have surgery, or be given medical treatment, or inflicts this condition on a child.

neurotransmitter   A specific chemical agent released by nerve cells. This chemical crosses a gap to stimulate or inhibit another nerve cell.

NSAID   Nonsteroidal, anti-inflammatory, over-the-counter, easily obtainable drugs such as aspirin, ibuprofen, Aleve, Tylenol, and the like.

oral allergy syndrome   A reaction of itching or tingling in the mouth after eating certain foods. This can occur in people allergic to certain pollens.

osmols   A term used to describe a situation in which a food-allergic person can breathe in raw, fresh, or cooked food substance molecules from the air, and have an allergic reaction in the lungs, throat, or nose.

ovalbumin and **ovomucoid**   Protein portions of the egg, and found in egg white.

peanut   A food in the legume family.

peristalsis   A ringlike contraction of the stomach and intestines that moves the food along in waves. The action starts in the mid-stomach area, in which the food is mixed with gastric juices.

pH   The symbol for the negative logarithm of the hydrogen ion concentration measured in moles per liter. A pH value of more than neutral is called alkaline or base, which is the opposite of acidic. A pH value of less than neutral is acid. Neutral is usually a pH of 7.

phagocytosis   A process whereby a single-celled organism protects itself by surrounding an invader and destroying it with chemicals inside the cell.

pollen count   Approximate measure of the concentration of all the pollen (or of one particular type, like ragweed) in the air in a certain area at a specific time. Pollen counts tend to be highest early in the morning on warm, dry, breezy days and lowest during chilly, wet periods.

prick-skin test   A test to determine if a patient is allergic to certain substances. A physician places a drop of the substance being tested on the patient's forearm or back and pricks the skin with a needle, allowing a tiny amount to enter the skin. If the patient is allergic to the substance, a wheal (mosquito-bitelike bump) will form at the site within about 15 minutes. Prick-puncture tests involve the epidermal layer of skin. Another name for this is cutis and is the superficial portion of the skin.

projectile vomiting   When emesis comes out in such force that the ejected food may virtually be shot across the room.

proteasis   Enzymes that break down protein.

pruritis   Itching.

pylorus   A part of the body where the food leaves the stomach.

pyrosis   Heartburn. Greek for "burning." The burning experience in heartburn is felt in the chest after eating.

Qi   Life energy, life force, and vital force within all nature.

RAST   A blood test that measures specific IgE. The letters stand for Radio labeled Allergo Sorbent Test.

reagin   An allergist's term for IgE antibodies.

receptor   A protein molecule on the cell surface or within the cell that binds to a drug, hormone, allergen, or neurotransmitter.

reflux   From the Latin meaning "backflow."

rennin   An enzyme that curdles milk.

respiratory system   A group of organs responsible for carrying oxygen from the air to the bloodstream and for expelling carbon dioxide.

rhinitis   An inflammation of the mucous membrane that lines the nose, often due to an allergy to pollen, dust, or other airborne substances. Seasonal allergic rhinitis is also known as "hay fever," a disorder that causes sneezing, itching, a runny nose, and nasal congestion.

sclerology A diagnostic method that interprets the shape and condition of blood vessels on the white membrane (sclera) of the eyeball. This method was developed by Native Americans.

seasonal allergic rhinitis Allergic reactions of the eyes, nose, and throat during certain months of the year.

second-generation antihistamines Nonsedating antihistamines.

serum The part of the blood without cells.

shellfish Fish without fins.

shiatsu Japanese art of healing, incorporating therapeutic massage, meditation, and self-healing to clear and balance the life force.

sinus (paranasal sinuses) Air cavities within the facial bones, lined by mucous membranes similar to those in other parts of the airways.

sinusitis An inflammation of the membranes lining the facial sinuses, often caused by bacterial or viral infection, or allergic reaction.

skin test A test in which an antigen is placed on the skin to see if there will be an IgE-related reaction.

soma From the Greek meaning "body." This refers to the axial parts of the body, such as the head, neck, and trunk.

specificity When an individual immunoglobulin is programmed to search out an antigen in its original form.

stunting Low height for age.

succussion A vigorous shaking after each dilution during the preparation of liquid homeopathic products. Proponents claim that this "releases energy" that "potentizes" the mixture for each dilution and that the process and outcome differ from that of ordinary serial dilution.

T cell A lymphocyte which undergoes a developmental stage in the thymus.

tolerance Diminished or absent capacity to make a specific response to an antigen, usually produced as a result of contact with that antigen under nonimmunizing conditions.

traditional Chinese medicine (TCM) Aims to strengthen the immune system to prevent discomfort, disorder, and disease. It says that Qi, vital energy, manifests both as yin and yang, and is present in all opposites, which are really inseparable.

tree nuts Nuts that are grown on trees.

up regulation   When the B memory cell makes multiple other B cells to produce the immunoglobulin.

urticaria   A skin condition, commonly known as hives, characterized by the development of itchy, raised white lumps or welts surrounded by an area of red inflammation.

vaccination   Originally referred to immunization against smallpox with the less virulent cowpox (vaccinia) virus; more loosely used for any immunization against a pathogen.

wasting   Low weight for age.

wheal   A tiny swelling in the skin where the fluid leaks out of the blood vessels into the tissue. Flare is the red area surrounding this wheal and occurs because the blood vessels have dilated.

wheat   A cultivated grass used as a food source.

white blood cell   Cells in the blood that help to protect the body against infection and invasion by foreign substances.

Zen-shiatsu   A form of therapy in which thumb and palm pressure is applied to the meridians.

Index

A

AAAAI (American Academy of Allergy, Asthma and Immunology), 193
AAFCO (Association of American Feed Control Officials), 157
AARP (American Association of Retired Persons), 185
acid in the stomach, 57
acid reflux, 57-58
acid sensitive esophagus, 60
acidophilus, 215
active chemicals in foods, 41-42
acupressure, TCM (Traditional Chinese Medicine), 239
acupuncture, TCM (Traditional Chinese Medicine), 238-239
additives, 172
adrenaline. *See* epinephrine
adverse effects
  acupuncture, 239
  herbs, 211
adverse reactions to food. *See* food intolerance
aflatoxin, 47
aging challenges, 142-149
  elderly persons and allergies, 147
    declining memory, 147
    laughter therapy, 149
    long-term care, 148
    recognizing stroke symptoms, 148
  management of allergies with existing conditions, 143
    analgesic use, 143
    asthma, 145-146

glaucoma, 144
incontinence, 144
infections, 144
itchy conditions, 144
topical nasal steroids, 143
  respiratory symptoms, 145
agricultural chemical, 46
air travel, 180-181
AK (Applied Kinesiology), 194
ALCAT (dubious diagnostic test), 194
alcohol, affect on the severity of medication side effects, 112
Alimentum, 136
alkaloids, 48
alkylamines (first-generation antihistamine), 109
Allegra (Fexofenadine), 111, 145
allergens, 10, 73
  cross-reactions, 79-80
  eggs, 74
  food families, 80-83
  major versus minor allergens, 72
  milk, 73-74
  peanuts, 75
  seeds, 78-79
  sensitization to, 5
  shellfish, 77
  tree nuts, 76-77
  true food allergies, 71-72
  wheat, 77
allergic reactions
  allergy-related facts, 5-9
  celiac disease, 78
  cross-reactions, plants, 11
  degranulation, 52
  dermatitis herpetaformis, 78
  food families, 80-83
  food-induced colitis, 78
  genetics, 7-8

immune system
  IgE-mediated immune system reactions, 21
  WBCs (white blood cells), 20, 51
medical conditions associated with food allergies, 10
most common foods, 10, 73
  cross-reactions, 79-80
  eggs, 74
  milk, 73-74
  peanuts, 75
  seeds, 78-79
  shellfish, 77
  soy, 76-77
  tree nuts, 76
  wheat, 77
nonceliac malabsorption, 78
outgrowing allergies, 34-35
process from sensitization to reaction, 21
role of lectins, 52
role of ricin, 52
sensitization to food allergen or protein, 5
signs and symptoms, 9-10
  anaphylactoid reaction, 32
  anaphylaxis, 30-33
  gastrointestinal reactions, 34
  oral allergy syndrome, 29-30
  respiratory reactions, 29
  skin reactions, 34
treatment options, 88
  alternative medicine, 89
  conventional medicine, 89
  environmental medicine, 89
  future research, 118-120
  medications, 107-117

6010